# BREAST CANCER

## The way to detection, protection and prevention

*by*

Dr Anita Khokhar

*An imprint of*

**B. Jain Publishers (P) Ltd.**
An ISO 9001 : 2000 Certified Company
USA — Europe — India

**BREAST CANCER**

First Edition: 2010
1st Impression: 2010

All rights reserved. No part of this book may be reproduced, stored in a retrieval system or transmitted, in any form or by any means, mechanical, photocopying, recording or otherwise, without any prior written permission of the publisher.

© with the author

Published by Kuldeep Jain for
**HEALTH HARMONY**
An imprint of
**B. JAIN PUBLISHERS (P) LTD.**
An ISO 9001 : 2000 Certified Company
1921/10, Chuna Mandi, Paharganj, New Delhi 110 055 (INDIA)
Tel.: 91-11-4567 1000 • Fax: 91-11-4567 1010
Email: info@bjain.com • Website: **www.bjainbooks.com**

Printed in India

ISBN: 978-81-319-0860-0

# Glossary

**Anatomy:** Normal structure of the body.

**Areola:** The area of dark coloured skin on the breast that surrounds the nipple.

**Aspirate:** Fluid withdrawn from a lump, often a cyst (for cyst see below).

**Axilla:** The underarm or armpit.

**Benign:** Not cancerous, does not invade nearby tissue or spread to other parts.

**Biopsy:** A procedure by which a portion of the lump is removed.

**Cervix:** Lower narrow portion of uterus where it joins with vagina.

**Cyst:** A sac or capsule filled with fluid.

**Estrogen:** Hormone maintaining female physical characteristics. It has a role to play in breast cancer.

**Excision:** To cut out or cut away.

**False negative:** Patients who have the disease but on tests show that they do not have the disease.

**False positive:** Patients who do not have the disease but on test show that they have the disease.

**Incision:** To make a cut.

**In situ:** In its original place.

**Lactation:** Breast feeding.

**Life style:** Way of life; It is composed of cultural and behavioral patterns and lifelong personal habits.

**Lymphatic system:** A system of vessels that carry waste from the cells in a fluid called lymph. The waste is filtered through lymph nodes which are distributed in groups throughout the body.

**Mammogram:** Breast X-ray.

**Mastectomy:** Surgical removal of a breast.

**Menarche:** Age of attaining puberty, when menstruation starts.

**Menopause:** Age when menstruation stops.

**Menstruation:** Discharge of blood from uterus usually at monthly intervals.

**Metastasis:** When the cancer cells break away from the primary tumor and spread into other organs of the body through the blood stream or the lymphatic system.

**Mortality:** Related to death.

**Nulliparous:** Women who have never borne children.

**Physiology:** Normal functioning of the body.

**Primary:** Original site which gets involved.

**Progesterone:** A hormone that helps to initiate and maintain pregnancy.

**Prognosis:** Forecast or likely course of disease or an illness.

**Puberty:** Period of sexual maturing.

**Risk:** Chance of danger.

**Screening:** The search for unrecognized disease by means of rapidly applied tests or examination in apparently healthy individuals.

**Stage:** A system to evaluate the advancement and severity of cancer. It takes into account the size of the tumor, the number and location of cancerous lymph nodes and whether the cancer has spread to other organs or tissues. It is important to know the stage of the disease to plan the treatment.

**Survival rate:** It is the number of survivors in a group (For example, of patients) studied and followed over a period (For example, a five year period).

**Tumor:** Is equated with neoplasm or new growth usually not considered to be of benign origin.

**Vessel:** Duct or canal holding or conveying blood or lymph.

# Preface

*The greatest discovery of my generation is that human beings can alter their lives by altering their attitudes of mind.*
— **William James**, US Psychologist

Over the last few decades cancer is assuming increasing importance in the developing countries. Breast cancer is also emerging as a cause for concern. Changing life-styles and behavioral patterns of women has made them more prone to cancer of the breast more so in the metropolitan cities than in the rest of the country. The implications of the disease are serious when measured in terms of family hardship, disablement, and loss of life. Developing countries are warned to take appropriate steps to avoid 'the epidemic' of such diseases likely to come with socio-economic and health development.

For early detection of Breast Cancer, Breast Self-Examination (BSE) is a technique, which is simple to perform, free of cost and after practice can be performed by the women themselves in the privacy of their homes, for those who have breast cancer or are related to it in any way there are many vital issues they need to learn about.

I hope that this book will empower women to fight against breast cancer.

Dr Anita Khokhar (MD)

# Acknowledgements

The valuable comments and suggestions given by the following are gratefully acknowledged.

1. Dr Chaudhary K., DDG (SG), Indian Council of Medical Research, New Delhi
2. Dr Parmar V., Assistant Surgeon, Breast Service, Dept. of Surgical Oncology, Tata Memorial Center, Mumbai
3. Dr Seth T., Assistant Professor, Institute Rotary Cancer Hospital, A.I.I.M.S., New Delhi
4. Dr Prabhakaran P. S., Director, Kidwai Memorial Institute of Oncology, Bangalore
5. Dr Reddy K. S., Member-Secretary, Pondicherry Regional Cancer Society, JIPMER
6. Dr Bhowmick K. T., Consultant, Head of the Department of Radiotherapy, Vardhman Mahavir Medical College and Safdarjang Hospital, New Delhi
7. Prof. Chaudhari S., Director, Rashtra Sant Tukdoji Regional Cancer Hospital, Nagpur
8. Dr Dua P., Consultant, Radiologist, Deewan Chand Satypal Aggrawal Imaging and Research Center, Delhi.
9. Prof. Karwasara R. K., Head of Dept. Surgical Oncology, PGIMS, Rohtak (Haryana)
10. Prof. Patnaik B. K., Director, Acharya Harihar Regional Cancer Center, Manglabag, Cuttack
11. Dr Rao B. N., Director, MNJ Institute of Oncology and Regional Cancer Center, Red Hills, Hyderabad
12. Prof. Seam K. R, Head Dept. of Radiotherapy and Oncology, Indira Gandhi Medical College, Shimla
13. Dr Shah S.V., Professor and Head, Dept. of Surgical Oncology, Gujarat Cancer and Research Institute (M.P. Shah Cancer Hospital)
14. Mr Devender Nayak, artist, Kala Kutir, Gardhi, New Delhi

## Publisher's Note

Today, breast cancer is a cause of global concern and this book, we are proud to say, is a well-seasoned expert's contribution towards outlining the steps to combat the disease. Despite pessimistic projections by world health bodies, the author lays stress on a problem-solving approach. The questions that increasingly trouble women as they confront the statistics on the disease are brilliantly answered, from health care and hospitalization to ways of preventing the disease.

For those who already are combating the disease or are in any way related to it, this book discusses the many vital issues they need to know about. Early detection is crucial and so is timely medical consultation.

It is important to note that increase in the population size and longer life expectancy are the two factors which have made the statistics on breast cancer seem so scary.

Let us devote our energies towards action, in order to bring about maximum benefit to maximum people, so that gradually women in the developing countries can lead healthier, sunnier and hopeful lives.

**Kuldeep Jain**
C.E.O., B. Jain Publishers (P) Ltd.

# Contents

*Glossary*   *iii*
*Preface*   *v*
*Acknowledgements*   *vii*
*Publisher's Note*   *viii*

1. Introduction .................................................................. 1
2. The Need for Breast Self Examination (BSE) ........................ 5
3. Breast Cancer and those at Risk ...................................... 9
4. Diet and Breast Cancer ................................................. 15
5. Anatomy, Physiology and Development of Breast ............... 31
6. Estrogen and the Risk of Breast Cancer ........................... 45
7. Types of Breast Cancer ................................................ 51
8. When and how to Perform Breast Self Examination (BSE) .... 59
9. How to Diagnose Breast Cancer ..................................... 71
10. Pregnancy and Breast Cancer ....................................... 75
11. Types of Treatment ..................................................... 91
12. Side Effects of Treatment of Breast Cancer ..................... 121
13. Evidence Based Management of Patients ....................... 143
14. Issues after Breast Cancer Treatment ........................... 153
15. What is Counseling? .................................................. 161
16. Recurrence of Breast Cancer ....................................... 173
17. Breast Cancer in Men ................................................. 181
18. Alternative Therapies for Breast Cancer Treatment .......... 189

*References*   201

Chapter 1
# Introduction

Breasts are a vital part of the human body and a source of interest to all. Not only do they add to the beauty of a woman's body but they also perform a vital function of breast feeding. But if a lady suffers from breast cancer then everything else becomes secondary. It becomes an all important issue of life over death. Therefore, it is essential that women look after the health of their breasts.

Breast cancer is one of the commonest causes of mortality in many developed countries in middle aged- women, and is becoming frequent in developing countries as well.[1] Breast self examination (BSE) is one screening technique by which a woman conducts a thorough examination of her entire breasts and armpits with the use of the fingers to check for any lumps that might have developed in these places. It has been observed that women themselves find most of the lumps. [2, 3]

## Global Scenario

Globally, the number of new cases of cancers was estimated to be 10.1 lakh in the year 2000. This represents a 20% increase over the previous decade. 53% of the cases occurred in the developing world. Similarly, 56% of the estimated deaths from cancers occurred in the developing world. The World Health Organization has forecast the cases to dramatically increase to 20 million by 2020. It is expected that 70% of the cases would occur in the developing world, which has access to only 5% of the global resources. [4]

The increase in number of cancer cases is not only due to an increase in the population size but also due to a dramatic increase in life expectancy.

Breast remains the leading area to be affected by cancer among women in the developed world. It is also the leading cause of death amongst them. In the year 2000, globally 10.5 lakh cases of breast cancer were reported. There were 3.73 lakh deaths and 38.6 lakh prevalent cases. By 2010 there are likely to be cases 11.45 lakh[5]. More than half of these cases are in the developed countries. When women migrate from low risk (developing countries) to high-risk (developed countries) regions, after two to three generations their descendants slowly acquire the rates of the host country. This illustrates the importance of lifestyle.[6] Cancer of the breast and cervix are the two most important cancer sites. They are responsible for one half of all the cases diagnosed in the women of the developing world.

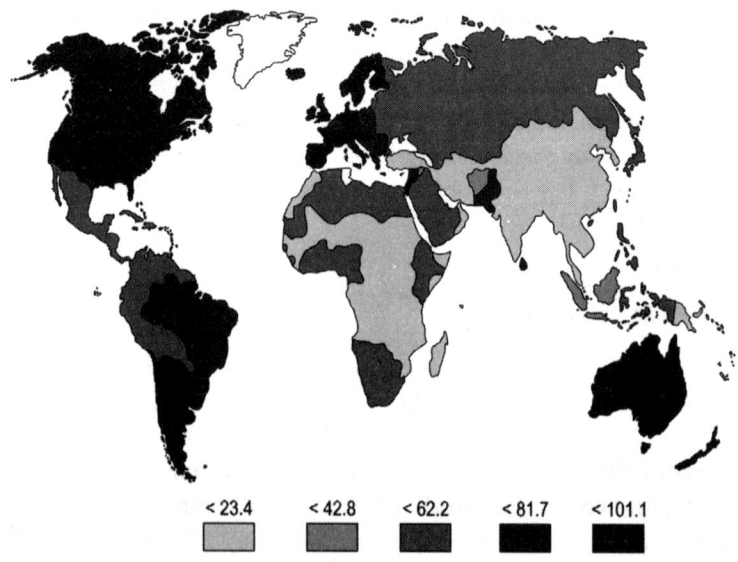

Breast cancer Incidence Rates per 100,000 worldwide according to GLOBOCAN, 2002 [7]

Breast Cancer Incidence and Mortality Rate per 100,000 by region or country. [8]

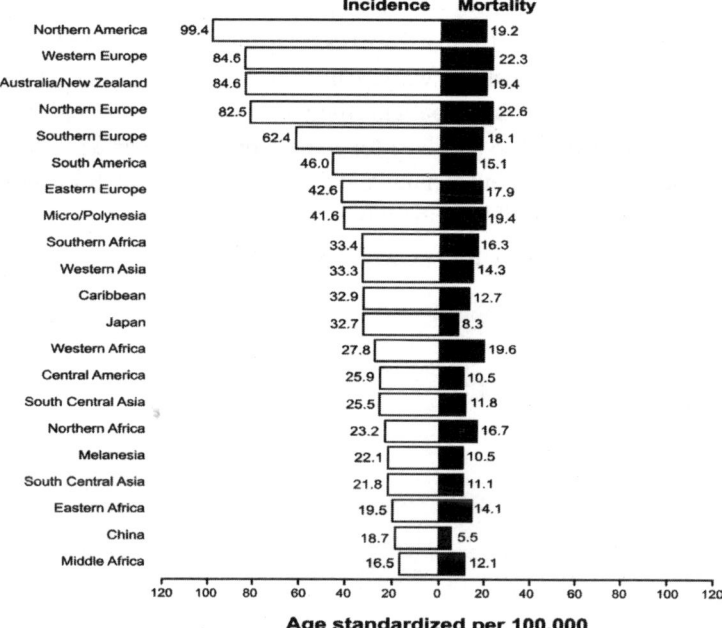

## Indian Scenario

It is estimated that there are nearly 2-2.5 lakh cases of cancer in the country at any given time. Nearly 8 lakh cases were diagnosed in the year 2000 and 5.5 lakh deaths due to cancer occurred in India.[4]

Among the Indian women, total number of cases of cancer of the breast and cervix are half of all the cancer cases. The Indian Council of Medical Research data shows that it is the commonest cancer to affect women in the cities of Delhi, Mumbai and Thiruvananthapuram[9]. Hospital Based Cancer Registry (1994-98) which includes all the patients treated by an institution whether in patients(admitted) or out patients shows that in Mumbai 26.2% and in Thiruvananthapuram 25.4% of the cancers in women were of breast. Cities of Bangalore, Chennai and Dibrugarh also show an increase in the cases of cancer of the breast. According to Population Based Cancer Registry (2001-

03) which covers the complete cancer situation in a given geographic area, cancer of breast contributed to 24.58% of the total cancers amongst women in Bangalore, in Delhi to 25.11%, Mumbai 27.47%, Chennai 26.07% and Bhopal 24.91%.[10] Both in Delhi and Mumbai rise in number commences at an earlier age.[11] The five-year relative survival (out of a group of patients diagnosed, treated and studied for 5 years those likely to survive) for female breast cancer was 46.8% in Bangalore, 49.5% in Chennai and 55.1% in Mumbai.[6] Soon there will be 90,000 to 1 lakh incident (new) cases annually.[12]

One in 22 urban Indian woman is likely to suffer from this disease.

Chapter 2

# The Need for Breast Self Examination (BSE)

## What is Breast Self-Examination (BSE)?

Breast self-examination (BSE) is when a woman uses her hands to systematically inspect her breasts and the surrounding areas for unusual lumps and shape changes. BSE is usually done on a regular basis, with the same technique each time. This technique ensures that all areas of the breast are felt and examined thoroughly. The purpose of BSE is to make a lady self aware and to screen for breast cancer and detect breast cancer as early as possible.[13,14] The breast examination can also be done by the male partner or spouse of the female.

Women frequently touch their own breasts while showering, dressing, having sex, etc. Some doctors urge women to touch their breasts often so that they know what their breasts normally feel like and can identify when unusual changes occur. However, BSE is different from simply touching your breasts and 'getting to know' your breasts. It is a method developed for the specific purpose of searching for cancer. Some people feel that this deliberate searching makes women overly anxious about breast cancer and unnecessarily fearful about every lump that they find. In some cases, this fear may eventually discourage women from touching their breasts. In the 1950s, Dr Cushman Haagensen, a breast surgeon at Columbia University, New York, noticed a disturbing trend. Women were coming to him with such large lumps which were inoperable. Haagensen discovered the

BSE application and encouraged his patients to examine themselves in order to find any lumps while they were still operable.[15]

In historical context the notion of BSE emanated from the theory – popularized by American surgeon William Halsted in the early 1900s – that breast cancer begins as a local disease that is more curable if discovered early.[16] One of its first proponents was New York physician Hugh Auchincloss, who in 1929 wrote that waiting for a lump to appear made little sense.[17] Ironically, among the strongest early advocates of BSE were Nazi health officials, who viewed the technique as a way to improve the health of Aryan women.[18] As it happened, it was the defeat of the Axis Powers in World War II that laid the groundwork for the popularization of BSE in the US. Having vanquished the Nazis, America turned its attention to the next enemy, cancer.[18]

In 1950, the American Cancer Society and the National Cancer Institute introduced a film, Breast Self-Examination, that was eventually viewed by more than 13 million women.[19] Accompanying educational material reiterated the point that finding smaller cancers by BSE dramatically improved a woman's chances of survival. Look magazine confidently reported that American women who performed BSE 'can virtually conquer the fatal aspects of this disease by their own initiative.'[20] By 1951, the Canadian Cancer Society was distributing American Cancer Society leaflets about BSE and generating its own material.[21]

The campaign to promote BSE played on traditional gender roles that placed special responsibility on women for guarding their health.[22] A woman who permitted a breast lump to grow, wrote one physician, 'has committed suicide almost as certainly as if she had blown out her brains with a pistol.'[23] Yet, whether imposed by society or embraced by women themselves, the duty to perform BSE took on special importance when advocated by a supposedly cured breast cancer patient. 'My life was saved,' one such woman wrote in 1955, 'because I practised breast self-examination.'[24] Even more powerful were accounts by women who stated that they were dying of breast cancer because they had never performed BSE. Although of questionable validity, such testimonials were hard to contradict.

# The Need for Breast Self Examination (BSE)

Breast self-examination received an additional push from the women's health movement, which emerged in the US, Canada and elsewhere in the 1970s.[16] BSE, like other healthful practices, became a mechanism for women to monitor the condition of their breasts and thus become less reliant on the medical system. When the American and Canadian cancer societies developed formal screening recommendations for breast cancer, they included BSE as well as annual breast examinations by health care professionals and screening mammograms. Efforts to promote mammography, like those to encourage BSE, have also conflated the seeming desirability of the test with its demonstrable value. For example, when the American Cancer Society began in the 1970s to recommend a baseline mammogram for healthy 35 year olds, one of its rationales was to instill 'good health habits' among women.[16]

About 80% of breast cancers not discovered by mammography are discovered by women themselves.[13] Some women find cancer during a breast self-exam; however, many women find cancer when they are touching or observing their breasts for other reasons. Breast cancer is also occasionally discovered when a woman's spouse or lover feels a lump inside.[13]

Early detection of breast cancer is of utmost importance for diagnosis of this disease. One benefit of the BSE lies in its potential to recognize and identify a breast lump while it is small and in early stage of development so that timely treatment can be initiated. All the women should be encouraged to perform BSE as more than 80% of the breast cancers are usually found by women themselves.

BSE can discover an early cancer in younger women in whom mammography is less effective.[25] Mammography for early detection has long been used as a screening tool in developed countries. It involves sophisticated imaging techniques, complex quality control procedures with enormous cost in terms of manpower and material resources. Further a larger proportion of such cancers occur in younger women in whom mammography is not a suitable approach for screening as their breasts are denser and more fibrous. One disadvantage of mammography is that it exposes a woman to radiation at a dose higher than that of an X-ray.[26]

If BSE technique is learnt correctly and practised monthly it could also be a useful tool for screening for interval cancers i. e. cancers which develop in between two mammography examinations.

Although results from a research conducted in Shanghai show that BSE does not reduce the number of women dying from breast cancer, what was also observed was that BSE did increase women's ability to find lumps which were of smaller size in their own breasts and definitely increased their awareness towards breast.[27] In a country like India, BSE will probably be the only feasible approach to wide population coverage for a long time to come as 50% of the women present themselves in late stages III and IV of the disease.[4] Further not only is there lack of health awareness even among educated but also hesitation to expose the breast due to socio- cultural influences.

BSE only takes a few minutes but it goes a long way towards increasing the familiarity of the women with their breasts so that they can notice any change, which is abnormal and also increases awareness about the disease.[28, 29] Thus the importance of the BSE must be impressed upon the women.

Chapter 3
# Breast Cancer and those at Risk

Cancer is regarded as a disease with following features:
i. Abnormal growth of cells.
ii. Ability to invade nearby tissues and even distant body organs.
iii. Eventual death of the affected person if the tumor has progressed beyond the stage when it can successfully be treated (that is, it has spread to many body organs).

## Who are the People at Risk?

1. **Age:** The risk of breast cancer increases as the woman gets older. It is uncommon before 20 years of age and thereafter its occurrence increases.

2. **Early menstruation and late menopause:** The influence of hormones like estrogen and progesterone are involved in onset of breast cancer.

3. **Late marriage and late full term pregnancy:** An early full time pregnancy seems to have protective effect. Women whose first pregnancy is delayed to their late thirties are at a higher risk than women who have borne many children.

4. **Genetic predisposition:** The risk of suffering from breast cancer increases if any of the family members (mother, sister, and daughter) have had breast cancer. The younger the family

member at the time of developing the cancer the greater the risk. Those with family history of bilateral (involving both the breasts) cancers are at an increased risk. Having genetic mutation in the breast cancer genes BRCA1 or BRCA2 also increases the risk.

5. **Socio-economic status:** It is more common in women from higher socio-economic groups because of affluent life style. Higher age at first childbirth and not breast feeding the child also increases the risk.

6. **Radiation therapy:** Women whose breasts are exposed to radiation under the age of 30 years are at a higher risk of developing cancer later in life.

7. **Diet, alcohol and smoking:** A diet high in fats, consumption of moderate amount of alcohol and smoking increases the risk.[30, 31]

8. **Obesity:** Weight gain as an adult or weight gain after menopause creates added risk. Higher levels of estrogen production in obese women probably have a role to play.[32]

9. **Personal history of breast cancer:** Women who have had cancer in one breast have an increased risk of getting it in the other breast.

10. **Oral Contraceptives and Hormone Replacement Therapy (HRT):** Combined hormone replacement therapy in Women's Health Initiative trial has shown the risk of breast cancer to increase.[33, 34]

11. **Race and ethnicity:** White women have higher incidence of breast cancer as compared to African and American women after the age of 40 years while African and American women have higher incidence before the age of 40. In contrast African and American women are more likely to die from breast cancer at all ages. Incidence and death rates are generally lower among women of other ethnic and racial groups than in white and African or American women.[35]

12. **Abnormal breast biopsy:** Some types of benign breast conditions are more closely linked to breast cancer risk than others. Doctors often divide benign breast conditions into 3 general groups,

depending on how they affect this risk: non-proliferative lesions, proliferative lesions without atypia, and proliferative lesions with atypia.[31]

**The proliferative lesions with atypia** (those with excessive growth of cells in the ducts or lobules of the breast tissue and the cells no longer appear normal) have a stronger effect on breast cancer risk, raising it 4 to 5 times higher than normal. They include:

 i. Atypical ductal hyperplasia (ADH)

 ii. Atypical lobular hyperplasia (ALH)

 iii. Women with a family history of breast cancer and either hyperplasia

 iv. Atypical hyperplasia have an even higher risk of developing a breast cancer.[31]

13. **Height adult:** Height is predictive of breast cancer risk. In international comparisons, height is positively correlated with breast cancer incidence rates. Both retrospective and prospective studies have frequently demonstrated clear associations between breast cancer risk and height. Recently, it has been postulated that height reflects the total number of ductal stem cells that develop in the breast in utero and thus the importance of prenatal exposures.[36]

14. **Chemicals:** Although risk factors are known to include the loss of function of the susceptibility genes BRCA1/BRCA2 and lifetime exposure to estrogen, the main causative agents in breast cancer remain unaccounted for. It has been suggested recently that underarm cosmetics might be a cause of breast cancer, because these cosmetics contain a variety of chemicals that are applied frequently to an area directly adjacent to the breast. The strongest supporting evidence comes from unexplained clinical observations showing a disproportionately high incidence of breast cancer in the upper outer quadrant of the breast, just the local area to which these cosmetics are applied. A biological basis for breast carcinogenesis could result from the ability of

the various constituent chemicals to bind to DNA and to promote growth of the damaged cells. Multidisciplinary research is now needed to study the effect of long-term use of the constituent chemicals of underarm cosmetics, because if there proves to be any link between these cosmetics and breast cancer then there might be options for the prevention of breast cancer.[37]

15. **Night shift work:** It has been proposed that exposure to light at night and power frequency (50–60 Hz) magnetic fields may increase the risk of breast cancer by suppressing the normal nocturnal production of melatonin by the pineal gland, which, in turn, could increase the release of estrogen by the ovaries. An increased risk of breast cancer was found among subjects who reported not sleeping during the period of the night when nocturnal melatonin levels are typically at their highest. This increased risk was found particularly among those subjects in the highest exposure groups. Breast cancer risk was also increased in subjects who reported working the graveyard shift at least some time in the 10 years leading up to a diagnosis of breast cancer, and there was clear evidence of a trend of increasing risk with increasing years of graveyard shift work and with more hours per week of work during the graveyard shift. No relationship was found between the risk of breast cancer and the number of times the subject reported getting up and turning on a light or the proportion of the night that this light was on. There was, however, some indication of an increased risk among subjects with the brightest bedrooms.[38]

16. **Lesbian:** The incidence of breast cancer among lesbians is unknown, although some studies claim that it is up to three times higher than in heterosexual women. Epidemiological evidence suggests that lesbians may be at greater risk for breast cancer; due to having fewer pregnancies and having children later in life, heavier alcohol consumption, higher body mass index and less access to prevention / treatment such as breast examinations by a physician. Lesbians, like women of colour and members of other oppressed groups, may also be at risk for late diagnosis and therefore greater mortality from cancer.[39]

17. **Flight attendants:** The increased risk of breast cancer and malignant melanoma among cabin attendants seems to be occupationally related. The part played by occupational exposures, i.e. cosmic radiation, disturbance of the circadian rhythm, and electromagnetic fields or combination of these factors in the etiology of breast cancer among the cabin crew, is still a puzzle as confounding due to parity appears to be ruled out. The relationship between the sunbathing habits of the cabin crew and the increased risk of malignant melanoma needs to be clarified. There is also an urgent need to elucidate the importance of these findings for today's aviation.[40]

Chapter 4

# Diet and Breast Cancer

## Role of Fats and Trans-fats in Breast Cancer

A diet high in fats has been often associated with breast cancer. Women's Health Initiative study of nearly 50,000 postmenopausal women across the United States provides first solid data on health effects of a low-fat diet. A low-fat diet was associated with a significant 15 percent reduction in estradiol, a form of blood estrogen that increases the risk of breast cancer.

Women in the low-fat group also experienced a 30 percent risk reduction for a certain subtype of breast cancer, tumors that were progesterone-receptor negative. Reducing dietary fat intake may decrease the chance of a breast cancer recurrence in women who have been treated for early-stage breast cancer, according to the Journal of the National Cancer Institute. Also high amount of fats in the diet are related with obesity which in turn is a high risk factor for breast cancer. We have been hearing a lot about the role of trans fatty acids in breast cancer. The increased risk of breast cancer appeared to be three and a half times as great among women with high intakes of trans fatty acids and low intakes of polyunsaturated fats (which come from fish and corn oils) compared to women who consumed significant amounts of polyunsaturated fat.

Analyzing tiny fat samples from 698 European women's buttocks revealed that those with breast cancer had higher levels of trans fatty acids stored in their bodies than women without breast cancer, according to a new international study. An increased intake of trans-fatty acids may raise the risk of breast cancer by 75 percent, suggest the results from the French part of the European Prospective Investigation into Cancer and Nutrition.[41, 42]

The study, the first to show a significant association between such fats and the life-threatening illness, is important because people can reduce trans fatty acid consumption by changing diets, researchers say. They suspect, but have not proven, that trans fatty acids may contribute to breast cancer development and that by cutting back on them, some women can protect themselves from the disorder.

Trans fat is the common name for a type of unsaturated fat with trans-isomer fatty acid(s). Unlike other dietary fats, trans fats are not essential. Unsaturated fats, found in such foods as avocados and olive and corn oils are heart healthy, but in the air they can go rancid by absorbing oxygen and then decompose. Manufacturers can stop this process by bubbling hydrogen (hydrogenation) through the fat at a high temperature in the presence of a catalyst like nickel and in the absence of oxygen.

Foods containing artificial trans fats formed by partially hydrogenating plant fats may contain up to 45% trans fat compared to their total fat.[41] Baking shortenings generally contain 30% trans fats compared to their total fats, while animal fats from ruminants such as butter contain up to 4%. Those margarines not reformulated to reduce trans fats may contain up to 15% trans fat by weight.[42]

It has been established that trans fats in human milk fluctuate with maternal consumption of trans fat, and that the amount of trans fats in the bloodstream of breast fed infants fluctuates with the amounts found in their milk. Reported percentages of trans fats (compared to total fats) in human milk range from 1% in Spain, 2% in France, 4% in Germany, and 7% in Canada.[43]

Trans fats are also found in shortenings commonly used for deep frying in restaurants. Since the parial hydrogenation leads to decreased rancidity and prolonged shelf life of the fat it finds favour with the producers. As fast food chains routinely use different fats in different locations, trans fat levels in products can have large variation. For example, an analysis of samples of McDonald's french fries collected in 2004 and 2005 found that fries served in New York

City contained twice as much trans fat as in Hungary, and 28 times as much trans fat as in Denmark (where trans fats are restricted). At KFC, the pattern was reversed with Hungary's product containing twice the trans fat of the New York product. Even within the US there was variation, with fries in New York containing 30% more trans fat than those from Atlanta.[44]

There is no adequate level, recommended daily amount or tolerable upper limit for trans fats. Despite this concern, dietary recommendations have not recommended the elimination of trans fat from the diet. This is because trans fat is naturally present in many animal foods in trace quantities, and therefore its removal from ordinary diets might introduce undesirable side effects and nutritional imbalances if proper nutritional planning is not undertaken. Recommended consumption of trans fatty acid should be as low as possible while consuming a nutritionally adequate diet.[45] The World Health Organization has tried to balance public health goals with a practical level of trans fat consumption, recommending in 2003 that trans fats be limited to less than 1% of overall energy intake.

## Red meat

Red meat refers to meat which is red-coloured when raw, while in nutritional terminology, it refers to meat from mammals. All meats obtained from 'livestock' are 'red meats' because they contain more of muscle protein than chicken or fish. While red meat is a good source of complete protein and iron, its regular consumption presents several health risks, largely due to the saturated fat content. Recent studies indicate that red meat could pose a notable increase in cancer risk. The findings from Harvard Medical School on women who ate more than one-and-a-half servings of red meat such as lamb, beef or pork, daily had almost double the risk of hormone receptor-positive breast cancer compared with those who ate three or fewer servings per week, the findings published in the journal Archives of Internal Medicine show.

Some studies have linked consumption of large amounts of red meat with breast cancer.[46] Women who ate more than 1½ servings of red meat per day were almost twice as likely to develop hormone-related breast cancer as those who ate fewer than three portions per week, one study found. In post-menopausal women it was a different story. Compared to eating no meat at all, even low levels of meat consumption were associated with a 52 per cent increased risk of breast cancer. High meat consumption was associated with a 63 per cent increased risk. This association was strongest for red and processed meat, hence the headlines. Poultry eating, on the other hand, was not significantly associated with risk of breast cancer in post-menopausal women. Processed meats, the report explains, are simply too dangerous for human consumption because they contain chemical additives that are known to greatly increase the risk of various cancers, including colorectal cancer, breast cancer, prostate cancer, leukemia, brain tumors, pancreatic cancer and many more.[47] Fresh meat is refrigerated and has a very short shelf life (just a few days, usually). It's usually packed in simple wrappers, with no fancy logos or color printing.

Processed meat has many ingredients and is usually packaged for long-term shelf life. These products almost always contain sodium nitrite, the cancer-causing chemical additive that meat companies use as a color fixer to turn their meat products a bright red 'fresh-looking' color. Processed meat products include:

- Bacon
- Sausage
- Pepperoni
- Beef jerky
- Deli slices
- Hot dogs
- Sandwich meat (including those served at restaurants)
- Ham
- Meat 'gift' products like Christmas sausages
- Meat used in canned soups
- Meat used in frozen pizza
- Meat used in kid's lunch products
- Meat used in ravioli, spaghetti or Italian pasta products

On top of these chemical additives, processed meats also contain saturated animal fat that is often contaminated with PCBs, heavy metals, pesticide residues and other dangerous substances. Cattle in the United States are treated with hormones to promote growth, which could also influence breast cancer risk.

## Vegetables

The number of servings of vegetables in a woman's daily diet makes a large difference in her risk of breast cancer. Women who eat a diet rich in vegetables have a lower incidence of breast cancer. Each daily serving of a colorful, or non-starchy, vegetable is associated with a 10% reduction in the risk of breast cancer–even after accounting for weight and other known risk factors for breast cancer.

In studies on both premenopausal women in New York and postmenopausal women in Athens, Greece, those who ate more than five servings of colorful vegetables a day had breast cancer only half as often as women who ate less than three servings a day. The possibility of cutting one's breast cancer risk by 50% or more is an extremely important finding.

The vegetables that appear to affect breast cancer risk are the so-called colorful vegetables–that is, non-starchy vegetables. Broccoli, cabbage, carrots, tomatoes, peppers, and dark leafy green vegetables all qualify. Potatoes and other starchy vegetables do not. As a rule, any vegetable that has a deep green, red, yellow, or orange color is rich in antioxidants and nutrients as well as fiber. Although researchers do not understand all the reasons why a diet rich in these vegetables decreases a woman's risk of breast cancer, the findings consistently show that they do. Each additional serving of fruit or fruit juice beyond the average. 1-2 servings of fruit a day is associated with a drop of around 8% in the risk of breast cancer. Research indicates that it is the fruits and vegetables themselves, with their natural package of nutrients that lower the risk of breast cancer. No individual nutrient has been identified as being responsible for the reduction in risk. How might vegetables and fruits influence the risk of breast cancer?

It is biologically feasible that vegetable and fruit consumption could affect breast cancer risk. There are several ways that the natural chemicals found in vegetables and fruits might help reduce the risk of breast cancer and other cancers. Some of the mechanisms are listed below:

- Stimulate cell differentiation and stop cell proliferation. Cell differentiation is the process by which a cell in the body becomes functionally mature. Differentiated cells have a low proliferation rate. Cancer arises largely from proliferating cells which are not differentiated. Compounds in vegetables and fruits, such as carotenoid-derived vitamin A, can encourage cells to differentiate and potentially protect against cancer formation.
- Act as antioxidants. Cells are exposed to oxidants from oxygen, some products of metabolism and from oxidant-producing toxins. Oxidants can damage various parts of cells including their DNA. Such damage can potentially lead to cancer formation. Vegetables and fruits contain many antioxidants, such as vitamin C and carotenoids. These chemicals can neutralize oxidants.
- Increase activity of protective detoxifying enzymes. Cells in the body are exposed to various toxins including cancer-causing compounds. These toxins can be deactivated and eliminated from the body by protective enzyme systems. Some chemicals in vegetables and fruits, such as dithiolthiones in broccoli, have been shown to increase the activity of the protective enzyme systems in the body.
- Enhance immune function. The consumption of vegetables and fruits may strengthen the immune system, which is the body's defense against various diseases including cancer.
- Alter estrogen levels. Estrogen is a hormone that is necessary for childbearing, but higher lifetime exposure to estrogen's actions is associated with higher breast cancer risk. Estrogen is normally metabolized to forms that have different strengths of action. Vegetables and fruits have compounds, such as glucosinolates in broccoli, that increase the metabolism of estrogen to weaker

forms. This effect may change the lifetime exposure to estrogen's actions and decrease breast cancer risk.
- Compete with naturally produced estrogen. Phytoestrogens, or plant estrogens, may be weaker than the estrogens which occur naturally in the body. The weaker phytoestrogens may compete with naturally occurring estrogens and block their effects (some of which are linked to breast cancer risk). However, some studies have raised concern that phytoestrogens may not be so weak, and they may increase rather than block estrogen activity.[48]

Women who eat four or more servings of fruits and vegetable per day have a 50 percent lower risk of breast cancer compared with women who eat two or fewer servings a day, according to a study presented by Oregon Health and Science University researchers[49] at the second annual Frontiers in Cancer Prevention Research meeting of the American Association for Cancer Research.

## Soy

Researchers believe phytoestrogens i.e. estrogens from plants found in soy may help protect against breast cancer because phytoestrogens compete with estrogen in the body to bind to estrogen receptors on cells. Since estrogen triggers breast cell reproduction, some researchers believe that a higher amount of estrogen in the body may increase a woman's risk for breast cancer. This is because phytoestrogens found in soy foods may block estrogen from reaching estrogen receptors, pre-menopausal women who include soy in their diet may decrease their risk of breast cancer. Though research on the effects of soy in pre-menopausal women shows some promise, it is preliminary and needs to be confirmed in large clinical trials.

Researchers are less certain about the effects of soy in post-menopausal women. Some small studies have shown that soy may provide post-menopausal women with many of the same benefits as hormone replacement therapy. Soy may reduce hot flashes, vaginal dryness, and other menopausal symptoms. Soy may also protect against bone loss (osteoporosis) and heart disease and possibly reduce the risk of diabetes and kidney disease. These estrogens from plant could possibly be misinterpreted by the body as estrogen and increase the risk of breast cancer in post-menopausal women. A variety of health benefits, including protection against breast cancer, have been attributed to soy food consumption, primarily because of the soybean isoflavones (genistein, daidzein, glycitein). Isoflavones are considered to be possible selective estrogen receptor modulators but possess nonhormonal properties that also may contribute to their effects. Concern has arisen over a possible detrimental effect of soy in breast cancer patients because of the estrogen-like effects of isoflavones. Many soy foods are rich in phytoestrogens, natural chemicals that act like weak estrogen (a hormone found in the female body). Isoflavones are one type of phytoestrogen. Isoflavones contain several compounds, including genistein and daidzin. Some researchers believe that isoflavones can alleviate menopausal symptoms and help prevent breast cancer in some women. Phytoestrogens are found in soybeans, flaxseeds, black cohosh, alfalfa spouts, and other plants.

Some physicians feel that women with estrogen receptor-positive breast cancers or those who are taking the drug tamoxifen for breast cancer should limit their intake of soy products containing phytoestrogens until researchers are able to better understand the effects of soy on breast tumors. In fact, many physicians advise women with a strong personal or family history of breast cancer not to consume phytoestrogens.

According to a Japanese report rather than protecting against all breast cancers, high levels of soy food consumption appears to specifically reduce the risk of estrogen receptor (ER)-positive tumors and human epidermal growth factor receptor 2 (HER2)-negative tumors.[50] More clinical trials are needed before we can clearly state the role of soy in breast cancer.

## Antioxidants

Antioxidants are substances or nutrients in our foods which can prevent or slow the oxidative damage to our body. When our body cells use oxygen, they naturally produce free radicals (by-products) which can cause damage. Antioxidants act as 'free radical scavengers' and hence prevent and repair damage done by these free radicals. Health problems such as heart disease, macular degeneration, diabetes, cancer etc are all contributed by oxidative damage. Indeed, a recent study conducted by researchers from London found that 5 servings of fruits and vegetables reduce the risk of stroke by 25 percent. Antioxidants may also enhance immune defence and therefore lower the risk of cancer and infection. Antioxidants are found in varying amounts in foods such as vegetables, fruits, grain cereals, legumes and nuts. Some antioxidants such as lycopene and ascorbic acid can be destroyed by long-term storage or prolonged cooking.[51, 52] Other antioxidant compounds are more stable, such as the polyphenolic antioxidants in foods such as whole-wheat cereals and tea.[53, 54] In general, processed foods contain fewer antioxidants than fresh and uncooked foods, since the preparation processes may expose the food to oxygen and oxidation of food, so food is preserved by keeping in the dark and sealing it in containers.

Antioxidants are abundant in fruits and vegetables, as well as in other foods including nuts, grains and some meats, poultry and fish. The list below describes food sources of common antioxidants.

i. Beta-carotene is found in many foods that are orange in colour, including sweet potatoes, carrots, cantaloupe, squash, apricots, pumpkin, and mangoes. Some green leafy vegetables including collard greens, spinach, and kale are also rich in beta-carotene.

ii. Lutein, best known for its association with healthy eyes, is abundant in green, leafy vegetables such as collard greens, spinach, and kale.

iii. Lycopene is a potent antioxidant found in tomatoes, watermelon, guava, papaya, apricots, pink grapefruit, blood oranges, and other foods. Estimates suggest 85 percent of American dietary intake of lycopene comes from tomatoes and tomato products.

iv. Selenium is a mineral, not an antioxidant nutrient. However, it is a component of antioxidant enzymes. Plant foods like rice and wheat are the major dietary sources of selenium in most countries. The amount of selenium in soil, which varies by region, determines the amount of selenium in the foods grown in that soil. Animals that eat grains or plants grown in selenium-rich soil have higher levels of selenium in their muscle. In the United States, meats and bread are common sources of dietary selenium. Brazil nuts also contain large quantities of selenium.

v. Foods rich in vitamin A include liver, sweet potatoes, carrots, milk, egg yolks and mozzarella cheese.

vi. Vitamin C is also called ascorbic acid, and can be found in high abundance in many fruits and vegetables and is also found in cereals, beef, poultry and fish.

vii. Vitamin E, also known as alpha-tocopherol, is found in almonds, in many oils including wheat germ, safflower, corn and soybean oils, and also found in mangoes, nuts, broccoli and other foods.

## Role of Pesticide and Dioxin in Breast Cancer

The role of pesticides in breast cancer is controversial. The debate generally focuses on studies that have, or have not, demonstrated a link between residues of DDT or its metabolite DDE in women, and increased risk of breast cancer.

Pesticides may increase Breast Cancer risk:

- Because they are mammary carcinogens, initiating cancer through mutations in a gene or causing other damage to DNA
- Because they are tumor promoters, and so promotes the growth of breast cancer cells and hormonally sensitive tumors
- By affecting mammary gland development in ways that increase susceptibility to carcinogens or hormonally active agents
- By compromising the immune system and reducing the body's defences against cancer
- By interfering with communication between cells, and hence also in the growth of tumors
- By disrupting the endocrine system in ways other than promoting tumors or affecting the development of mammary gland tissue (see below)

- Other mechanisms may also be involved; intrauterine growth retardation has been shown to increase susceptibility in later life to breast cancer.

After taking into account other known risk factors for breast cancer, the researchers write that the risk of breast cancer was twice as high in women with the highest (blood) concentrations of dieldrin (an organ chlorine) as that in women with the lowest concentrations.[55]

## Interference with hormones

Hormonally active pesticides not only enhance breast cell proliferation but can also play critical roles in the development of breast cancer. There is strong evidence from laboratory tests that estrogen-mimicking chemicals promote the growth of human breast cells.

- there are critical periods of rapid breast cell proliferation during which the breast is more vulnerable to the influence of chemicals, and at these times exposure to even extremely low doses can cause permanent damage - prenatal, early childhood, menarche, first childbirth and perimenopause.

No pesticide can be claimed to not cause breast cancer until the mechanisms summarised here have been fully explored for each pesticide.

## Dioxins

Of all toxic chemicals, dioxins may be the most widespread. The body fat of every human being, including every newborn, contains dioxins. Dioxins are formed by the incineration of products containing PVC, PCBs and other chlorinated compounds; as well as from industrial processes that use chlorine, such as pulp and paper manufacturing; and from the combustion of diesel and gasoline. Dioxins break down very slowly; they accumulate in fat of wildlife and bioaccumulate across the food chain. People are exposed to dioxins primarily through consumption of animal products and human breast milk. Dioxin enters the food chain when vehicle exhaust or soot from incinerated chlorinated compounds falls on field crops later eaten by farm animals. It is then passed to humans through dairy and meat products.

There has been limited research examining possible effects of dioxin exposure and breast cancer risk.

However, a recent follow-up study on women exposed to dioxins during a chemical plant explosion in 1976 in Seveso, Italy makes a more compelling case for a connection between dioxin and breast cancer. Scientists analysed blood samples taken and stored at the time of the explosion and correlated the results with subsequent cases of breast cancer. They found that a tenfold increase in the levels of these was associated with more than twice the risk of breast cancer. Women who were children at the time of the accident are just beginning to reach the age when breast cancer is most likely to develop and researchers will continue to follow the Seveso women. They expect to find additional breast cancer cases.[56]

## Nicotine

When it comes to cancer, nicotine and cigarette smoking can increase your risk of cancer in general. The chemicals found in cigarettes are carcinogenic, or cancer causing. So smoking increases your risk of many types of cancer. Nicotine may spur the spread of breast cancer, pushing cells from the original tumor to other parts of the body, said a study published in the latest issue of Cancer Research, a journal of the American Association for Cancer Research.

Although scientists need time to pinpoint the exact role nicotine may play in breast cancer's spread, there is no doubt that nicotine may contribute to the metastasis that so often kills patients. Besides serving as yet another warning against smoking, the finding may also point to new targets for cancer drugs, Much of the past research on nicotine has been on the human nervous system, but recent studies have demonstrated that the chemical can also trigger signaling systems in non-neuronal cells, including cancer cells. 'It has been known that there are 10 to 12 nicotine receptors that express on the surface of various cells. When nicotine is attracted to these receptors and binds there, they begin "telling" the cells to grow in the out-of-control fashion that defines cancer. And, once the cells are cancerous, the receptors tell them to migrate to distant parts of the body through the bloodstream, a process known as metastasis.' Yet nicotine didn't seem to be able to accomplish this on its own. Nonetheless, the study couldn't identify which other factors might be assisting nicotine in the cancer scenario. This portion of the study was done in the test tube, but Chen reproduced the findings in mice.[57]

## Alcohol

Alcohol may change the way the body metabolizes estrogen. Many breast cancers are fuelled by the hormone estrogen. Therefore, regular use of alcohol is thought to increase the risk of breast cancer by increasing blood estrogen levels.

A new study tracked the health of 122,000 women since 1976. They were free of cancer at the start of the study. Every four years, the women were asked how much alcohol they had used during an average month in the past year.

By 2002, nearly 6,000 of the women developed breast cancer.

When compared with teetotalers:

- Women who drank the equivalent of a half glass of wine a day were 6% more likely to develop breast cancer.
- Women who drank a glass or two a day faced a 21% increased risk of breast cancer.
- Those who drank more than two drinks a day were 37% more likely to develop breast cancer.

However, the risk was much greater in menopausal women:

- Menopausal women who drank half a glass of wine daily increased their chance of breast cancer by 18%.

The elevated risk was also more pronounced for women whose tumor growth was fuelled by the hormones estrogen or progesterone-- a group that accounts for about 70% of women with breast cancer. Overall, moderate drinking raised the risk of developing breast cancer, regardless of whether a woman's preference was for beer, wine, or hard liquor. And the more she drank, the greater the risk.

Drinking as little as half a glass of wine a day may raise a woman's risk of developing breast cancer, a new study shows.[58]

The study found that those who had less than one drink a day (14gms alcohol) had a 7% increased risk for breast cancer compared to those who did not drink at all. Two drinks a day increased the risk by 32% (28 gms of alcohol). Women who drank three or more glasses of alcohol each day had a 51% higher risk.

## How can Physical Activity Reduce Breast Cancer Risk?

The association of physical activity with breast cancer incidence has been extensively studied with over 60 studies published in North America, Europe, Asia and Australia. Most studies indicate that physically active women are at lower risk of developing breast cancer than inactive women; however the amount of risk reduction achieved through physical activity varies widely (between 20-80%).[59, 60] While most evidence suggests that physical activity reduces breast cancer risk in both premenopausal and postmenopausal women[59], high levels of moderate and vigorous physical activity during adolescence may be especially protective. Although a lifetime of regular, vigorous activity is thought to be of greatest benefit, women who increase their physical activity after menopause may also experience a reduced risk compared to inactive women. A number of studies also suggest that the effect of physical activity may be different across levels of BMI, with the greatest benefit seen in women in the normal weight range (generally a BMI under 25 kg/m-square) in some studies. Existing evidence shows decreasing risk of breast cancer as the frequency and duration of physical activity increases. Most studies suggest that 30-60 minutes per day of moderate-to high-intensity physical activity is associated with a reduction in breast cancer risk.[59, 61] Researchers have proposed several biological mechanisms that may explain the relationship between physical activity and breast cancer development. Physical activity may prevent tumor development by lowering hormone levels, particularly in premenopausal women, lowering levels of insulin and insulin-like growth factor I (IGF-I) improving immune response, and assisting with weight maintenance to avoid a high body mass and excess body fat.[61] According to British Journal of Sports Medicine physically active women are 25 per cent less likely to get breast cancer, Physical activity reduced breast cancer risk in all women except the obese and had the greatest impact in lean women (BMI < 22kg/m$^2$). [62]

Chapter 5

# Anatomy, Physiology and Development of Breast

Breasts are that part of the body which is well developed in women as compared to men. Although the development of breast starts before birth it is only after puberty that they develop completely under the influence of ovarian hormones and hormones of pregnancy. The shape of the breast also changes as one grows older. They become more droopy.

## Structure

One way to visualise the structures of the breast is to picture a tree. The alveoli are the leaves and the ducts are the branches. Many smaller branches merge into a few bigger branches that finally become the trunk of the tree. Similarly, the breast is made up of units called lobes, each one composed of a single major duct with multiple smaller ducts and alveoli leading into it. Most authorities believe that women have approximately 15 to 20 lobes per breast.

Within each lobe there are many smaller lobules. Lobules end in dozens of tiny bulbs that produce milk. The lobes, lobules and bulbs are all linked by thin tubes called ducts. These ducts lead to the nipple in the centre of a dark area of skin called areola. Fat surrounds the lobules and the ducts. There also are body hairs on the breast, and they may be especially prominent in the areolar area. Their presence is normal and does not indicate masculinity. The size of the breast and the number and colour of the hair is determined by the genetic make up of a person.

Ligament of Cooper anchors the skin and the gland to the underlying pectoralis muscle. Infiltration of these ligaments by cancer cells causes fixity of the gland and puckering (wrinkling) of the skin.

**Axillary tail** is extension of the breast in to the armpit. It can be felt in a few normal individuals, during pre-menstrual period and during lactation. A well-developed axillary tail may be mistaken for enlarged lymph nodes (which are involved in the cancer of breast). Each breast also contains blood vessels and lymph vessels. The lymph vessels drain lymph, and lead to small structures called lymph nodes. Clusters of lymph nodes draining the breast lie in the axilla (under the arm), above the collarbone, in the chest and in many other parts of the body.

Cancers of the breast arise in the ductal and glandular structure. Most commonly involved part of the breast is the upper - outer quadrant.[63]

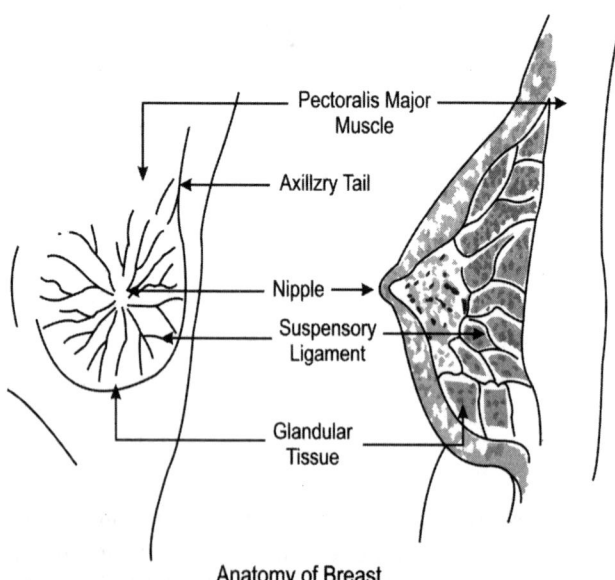

Anatomy of Breast

# Breast Development [64]

## Infancy

Breast development begins already in the womb, in both male and female foetuses. Between the fourth and seventh week of the embryo's life, the outer layer of the skin begins to thicken along a line extending from the armpit to the groin. This forms the mammary ridge. Later, most of this 'milk line' fades away, but a small portion remains in the chest and forms 16 to 24 buds that develop into milk ducts and alveoli, the sacs that secrete and store milk in the breast. This first stage of development begins at about six weeks of foetal development with a thickening called the mammary ridge or the milk line. By six months of development this extends all the way down to the groin, but then regresses. At this time, solid columns of cells form from each breast bud, with each column becoming a separate sweat gland. Each of these has its own separate duct leading to the nipple. By the final months of foetal development, these columns have become hollow, and by the time a female infant is born, a nipple and the beginnings of the milk-duct system have formed.

A secretion can be seen from the breasts of newborn babies. It is caused by the excessive hormones in the mother's blood which pass through the placenta and reach the fetus. The mammary glands then remain inactive until puberty.

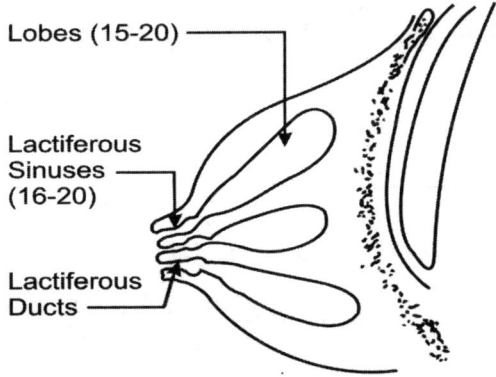

Lobes of the Mammary Gland

The breasts start to grow a year or two before a girl begins to menstruate. During each ovulatory cycle, the breast tissue grows a little more. Most growth occurs in adolescence, until a woman gives birth and begins to produce milk her breasts are not considered mature.[65] The American Cancer Society considers the human breast to be that area which extends from the center of the sternum (breast bone) downward to the 'bra line' (under the breasts), across to the side of the body, up to the center of the armpit (axilla), and across the clavicle (bone) to the top of the sternum (breast bone). This entire area should be carefully checked when doing a Breast Self Examination.

## Puberty

As a girl approaches adolescence, the first outward signs of breast development begin to appear. When the ovaries start to secrete estrogen, fat in the connective tissue begins to accumulate causing the breasts to enlarge. The duct system also begins to grow. Usually the onset of these breast changes is also accompanied by the appearance of pubic hair and hair under the arms.

Once ovulation and menstruation begin, the maturing of the breasts begins with the formation of secretory glands at the end of the milk ducts. The breasts and duct system continue to grow and mature, with the development of many glands and lobules. The rate at which breasts grow varies greatly and is different for each young woman.

# Female Breast Developmental Stages [66]

### Tanner stage 1 (ages 8-11)

The preadolescent breast consists of a small elevated nipple with no significant underlying breast tissue. The breast is just beginning to develop.

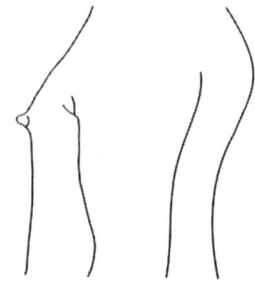

## Tanner stage 2 (ages 8-14)

Puberty begins usually between ages of 8 and 13, though the average age is 11, with the development of breast tissue and pubic hair. With the hormonal changes of puberty, breast buds form. This second stage of breast development is the breast bud stage. Here, there is elevation of the breast and nipple as a small mound; the areola begins to enlarge. Milk ducts inside the breast begin to grow.

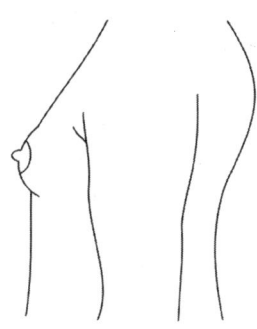

## Tanner stage 3 (ages 9-15)

In stage 3, there is further enlargement and elevation of the breast and areola (with no separation of their contours) The areola begins to darken in color. The milk ducts give rise to milk glands that also begin to grow.

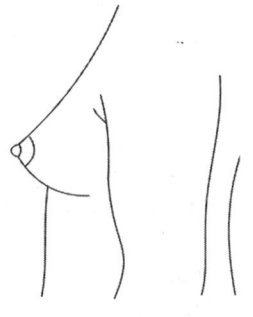

## Tanner stage 4 (ages 10-16)

Next, there is projection of the areola and nipple to form a secondary mound.

## Tanner stage 5 (ages 12-19)

In the mature adult breast, (were the breast is fully developed) there is a projection of the nipple only; however, in some woman the areola continues to form a secondary mound.

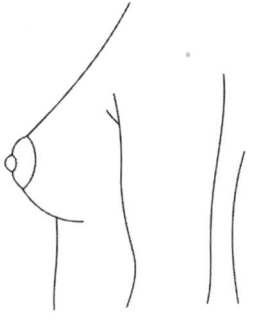

Each month, women experience fluctuations in hormones that make up the normal menstrual cycle. Estrogen, which is produced by the ovaries in the first half of the menstrual cycle, stimulates the growth of milk ducts in the breasts. The increasing level of estrogen leads to ovulation halfway through the cycle, and then the hormone progesterone takes over in the second half of the cycle, stimulating the formation of the milk glands. These hormones are believed to be responsible for the cyclical changes such as the swelling, pain, and tenderness that many women experience in their breasts just before menstruation.

During menstruation, many women also experience changes in breast texture, with breasts feeling particularly lumpy. These are the glands in the breast enlarging to prepare for a possible pregnancy. If pregnancy does not occur, the breasts return to normal size. Once menstruation begins, the cycle begins again.

The areola is the area of skin that surrounds the nipple. It is usually a different colour than the skin colour on the breast, and may vary from slightly darker than the skin to a very dark... nearly black. The colour is usually determined by the colour of the skin on the body, or the ethnicity of the person, and it will change during a person's lifetime. As women sexually mature and also when they become pregnant, the areola usually darken. After breastfeeding is completed, they may return to nearly the same colour as before the pregnancy. Their size can be as small as an inch across to several inches wide. They may even be wide enough to cover half the breast, although this is unusual. They will get wider during pregnancy, partly because the breast itself is enlarging.

A number of small bumps that surround the nipple and look like 'goose bumps' are sebaceous glands, and are called Montgomery's Glands or Areolar Glands. They secrete an oily substance that lubricates and conditions the surface of the nipple and the areola. This is helpful during breastfeeding, to prevent cracking of the nipple. These Montgomery's glands become erect when stimulated by touch, cold, fear, sexual stimulation, etc. like the nipples. Very small smooth muscle tissues cause them to become more prominent (erect). This also causes the areolar tissue to become narrower, but sexual stimulation will temporarily expand the breast itself.

Nipples have as many as 15 to 25 pores, one for each lobule in the breast. Nipples may be classified by their shape. If they come forward from the breast, they are considered to be prominent. They may also be flat, where they seem to be at the same level as the areola. Sometimes they may actually be depressed into the breast i.e. 'inverted' nipples. Be aware of how they are and pay close attention when you do a Breast Self Exam. Any way that they are is okay, but be concerned if they CHANGE. Check out the Breast Self Exam section for more information on this matter. No matter what the nipple is like (flat, inverted or prominent), the shape will not prevent you from breast feeding your child.

There are people who like to pierce their nipples. Consider waiting until after your breastfeeding years to do the piercing. Some nipples are exceptionally wide and some are exceptionally long, but some people attempt to modify their appearance by using various pieces of 'jewelry' that stretches them or enlarges them. Use care and common sense when making decisions about modifying your body.

**Parenchyma** is the term that describes breast tissue that is involved in the production or transporting of breast milk. This includes the lobes, which are the glands in which the milk is actually produced from the mother's blood. Sometimes referred to as alveoli or acini, these lobes are clustered on the ducts in a way that resembles grapes on the vine. When the brain signals the lobes to produce milk, it is gathered together by the lactiferous ducts and brought to the nipple area (lactiferous sinus). About two-thirds of the average pre-menopausal breast is parenchymal tissues. The amount of this tissue that is in the breast will not change when the person gains or loses weight but the amount of fatty tissue in the breast will change. The size of the breast will not necessarily determine the quantity of milk that a woman will produce. Smaller sized breasts are usually as successful at breastfeeding as larger ones. When a woman is pregnant, the lobes develop to the point that they can produce milk. That is why the breast enlarges during pregnancy, and is the reason women (and also men) do not normally produce milk until they have gone through a pregnancy.

Just before each lactiferous duct reaches the nipple, it swells out a little, creating what is called an ampulla (lactiferous sinus). This is the only part of the breast that actually holds a reserve of milk. This milk provides an enticement to the infant, to keep it at the nipple, while the lobes start the production of more milk. The ampullae are what need to be compressed when an infant (or the woman herself) wants to express milk from the breast. The infant has a little assistance by using suction.

Parenchyma, and a little of the stroma (non-milk bearing tissue) make up the density (or the firmness) of the breast. At about the age of 35 years, the breast becomes a little less dense. This is why mammograms are not usually done until after that age. Dense breast tissue makes it difficult to see signs of breast cancer on an x-ray film.

**Stroma** is the term used for breast tissue that does not deal with milk production. Muscle tissue, connective (Cooper's) ligaments and fatty tissue are included in this category. Men and woman have breasts. Just about anything that you will find in a female breast will be found in a male breast, but some of the components will be undeveloped in the male. Men (and that includes prepubescent and pubescent males) do not expect to see any breast development on their body, unless they put on a lot of fatty deposits or they build up some fantastic 'pecs' as a result of muscular development behind the breast (pectoralis muscles), and should not be confused with breast development. Women who exercise to increase their breast size merely increase the pectoral muscle size, which makes their chest wall measurement (above the breasts) larger. Their cup size does not change, unless they work really hard developing those pecs. Unfortunately, the change will most likely be a reduction in the cup size. Exercising muscles to develop them requires energy that may come from the burning of fatty deposits in the body, and those deposits may be those in the breasts.

Females may secrete a small amount of fluid from their nipples anytime after their breasts mature (and she is not pregnant or lactating). Be alarmed only if there is a sudden change in amount expressed, or its colour, or if one side suddenly is different than the other side.

A large number of males will have some breast swelling during their puberty. Although this panics the males it is usually a temporary situation that exists for less than a year and a half. Estradiol is produced from testosterone in male puberty as well as female, and male breasts often respond to the rising estradiol levels. This is termed gynecomastia. In most boys, the breast development is minimal, similar to what would be termed a 'breast bud' in a girl, but in many boys, breast growth is substantial. It usually occurs after puberty is underway, may increase for a year or two, and usually diminishes by the end of puberty. It is increased by extra adipose tissue if the boy is overweight.

Although normal breast development is usually unwelcome in boys and can be removed surgically if the boy's distress is substantial. A call to his doctor should alleviate any concerns that anyone may have.

Males should be as aware of their breasts as females should be of theirs. Males can get breast cancer. Any unusual changes to the skin or the interior of the breast or emissions from the nipple should be brought to the attention of their doctor.

We need to understand that there is nearly NO MUSCLE TISSUE in the breast. Exercise will not increase the size of the breast, because there are no muscles to develop. The pectoral muscles behind the breasts can be developed, which might push the breasts forward a little more, if the muscles are developed extensively. That much exercise, however, may result in the loss of body fat, and some of it may come from the breasts, making the breasts smaller than they were before the exercise program began. The exercise may be very healthy for you, though. There are some very minute muscles in the areola that cause an erection of the nipple and the Montgomery's glands. There are some tiny muscles around the lobules that help to express the milk, but there are no other muscles in the breast.

We all know what the fatty tissue does. It makes things bigger. The average sized breast of a pre-menopausal woman is about one-third fatty tissue. Larger breasts usually have more fatty tissue, but not more lobular tissue. Fatty tissue helps to fill out the voids and lumps of our bodies, and so it helps us to look softer, and smoother. The average woman has a higher percentage of body fat, so she will usually have a more rounded softness to her body, softer in appearance as well as touch.

Inside the breast, connecting the back-side of the breast skin to the pectoral muscles, are ligaments that make up what is called connective tissue. The ligaments are called Cooper's Ligaments, or Suspensory Ligaments. Their purpose is to provide the shape of the breast. They pull in on the skin, while the fatty tissue and the lobules press outward.

## Pregnancy and Lactation [67]

The hormones of pregnancy, including estrogen, progesterone, prolactin, and others, cause complex changes to occur in the breast. The various hormones each play a specific part in preparing the body for breastfeeding. However, enlargement is what women notice first of all. During the first trimester of pregnancy, the ducts and alveoli in the breast multiply rapidly. The breasts may be tender, and their size increases in preparation for breastfeeding.

**Lactogenesis** is the term denoting the origin, or the beginning, of lactation, and it occurs in three stages. Lactogenesis I starts at about 12 weeks before delivery, as the mammary glands begin to secrete colostrum. Breast size increases further as the alveoli become filled with colostrum, but the presence of high levels of the hormone progesterone in the mother's blood inhibits the full production of milk until after birth.

Lactogenesis II begins after birth when the placenta is delivered. Progesterone levels fall while prolactin levels remain high. Prolactin is the main hormone in charge of lactation, and it, in turn, is controlled by hormones secreted by the pituitary, the thyroid, the adrenal glands, the ovaries, and the pancreas. More blood flows to the breasts, carrying more oxygen. Two to three days postpartum, the 'milk comes in.' The amount of milk produced increases rapidly, and its composition gradually changes from colostrum to mature milk. Sodium chloride, and protein levels in the milk decrease and levels of lactose and other nutrients increase. The colour gradually changes from the golden yellow typical of colostrum to a bluish white. Since this process is controlled by hormones, the breasts begin to produce milk whether a mother is breastfeeding or not. At this stage of lactogenesis, it is important to breastfeed often (and/or pump, if the baby cannot feed well), because frequent breastfeeding in the first week after birth seems to increase the number of prolactin receptors in the breast. A receptor's job is to recognize and respond to a specific hormone. Having more prolactin receptors makes the breast more sensitive to prolactin, which researchers believe affects how much milk a mother produces in the next stage of lactogenesis.

Stage III of the lactogenesis process is characterised by continued milk production from now on which depends more on the ongoing removal of milk from the breasts than on the hormones circulating in the blood. The 'supply and demand' principle takes over. The more a mother nurses, the more milk she will produce. If she nurses less, milk production will slow down.

## Physiology and milk supply [67, 68, 69, 70]

Understanding how milk production works can help a mother ensure that her baby is getting enough milk at the breast. For example, sometimes mothers feel that their baby has completely emptied their breast and that there is no more milk available, even though the baby wants to nurse. Knowing that new milk is constantly being produced in the alveoli will give a mother the confidence she needs to put her baby to the breast, even when it feels 'empty' Breast feeding the child seems to offer protection against breast cancer.

Emptying the breasts is what keeps milk production going. A baby's sucking sends messages to the brain, which then releases the hormone oxytocin. Oxytocin causes the muscle cells around the alveoli to contract, pushing milk down through the ducts to the nipple. Mothers may experience it as a tingling feeling or a sense of release in the breast which is why it is also called the 'let-down.'

Another consideration related to milk supply is the breasts' storage capacity. Sometimes small-breasted women worry that they may not be able to make enough milk for their babies, but the milk production process makes adjustments for breast size. Smaller breasts may not be able to store as much milk between feedings as larger breasts, but if they are emptied often enough, they will make as much milk as the baby needs. Women with larger breasts and greater storage capacity may be able to go longer between feedings without affecting their supply. On the other hand, women with smaller breasts may need to nurse more frequently since their breasts fill faster and milk production slows down as the alveoli become full. Frequent nursing is not only good for supply, but it is also a healthy habit that helps mothers avoid plugged ducts and breast infections. Healthy babies with good breastfeeding skills take as much milk as they need when they need it, without mothers giving much thought to the whole process. But knowing how the whole process works can help a mother solve any problems she may be having with milk supply. It can also help her think through some of the myths and misunderstandings people have about breastfeeding. For example, she will know that she doesn't have to wait for her breasts to 'fill up' between feedings. There is always milk there for the baby. She will also know that if her baby seems hungry or is going through a growth spurt, nursing more often will speed up her milk production almost instantly

When someone takes medication or eats food, the substance is usually broken down by the digestive tract and then gets absorbed into the blood. When these molecules get to the capillaries near the breast tissue, they move through the cells that line the alveoli and into the milk, a process known as diffusion.

This is how ingredients needed to make milk get into the milk, as well as how drugs and other foreign substances enter milk. But many factors influence whether or in what quantity a substance will actually enter the milk. In the first days after birth, there are gaps between the lactocytes, the cells that line the alveoli and either block or allow substances to enter. These gaps mean that substances pass rather freely into the milk in the first days of life. After a few days, the gaps close. From then on, it is harder for substances to cross the barrier between the blood and the milk.

The process of diffusion allows good things, such as antibodies, to easily enter colostrum and mature milk. All women transfer antibodies to their babies during pregnancy and birth, but breastfeeding prolongs the time in which the mother's body helps protect the baby from illness.

Medications the mother takes may also get into her milk by crossing from blood through the lactocytes into the alveoli.

## After childbirth

Levels of estrogen, progesterone and other hormones fall sharply after childbirth causing a number of physical changes. The womb shrinks back to its non-pregnant size, pelvic floor muscle tone improves and the volume of blood circulating round the body returns to normal. The dramatic changes in hormone levels might also play a part in causing postnatal depression. It may be that some women are more easily affected by these hormonal fluctuations than others.

Talking of hormonal fluctuations, although they have been the subject of study for many years, we still don't know whether they are responsible for the wide range of physical and psychological symptoms we now call premenstrual syndrome or PMS. No-one doubts that many women experience tender breasts, abdominal bloating, irritability, low mood and other symptoms in the lead up to a period but whether these are due to hormone fluctuations, changes in brain chemicals, social and emotional problems or a combination of all three is a matter of debate.

## The menopause

The next significant hormonal change for most women occurs around the time of the last period - the menopause. Over three to five years leading up to a woman's last period, the normal functioning of her ovaries begins to change. This can cause menstrual cycle to become erratic. Periods may become heavier or lighter. Eventually, the ovaries produce so little estrogen that the lining of the womb fails to thicken up and so periods stop altogether.

For most of a woman's life, estrogen helps to protect the heart and bones, as well as maintaining the breasts, womb, vagina and bladder in their healthy state. The marked loss of estrogen in a woman's body that occurs around, and after, the menopause can, therefore, have detrimental effects on her health; as well as causing uncomfortable symptoms such as hot flushes and night sweats, lack of estrogen can increase the risk of heart disease and the bone disorder osteoporosis. Other problems include vaginal dryness, discomfort during sex, recurrent urine infections and incontinence. It may also contribute to the depression, irritability and poor concentration, which some menopausal women experience. If reduced, hormone levels do cause unpleasant symptoms, treatments such as hormone replacement therapy (HRT) are often very effective. HRT and other types of medication can also be used to prevent health problems, for example if a woman has a significantly increased risk of developing osteoporosis or heart disease in the future.

So, from the womb to the tomb, hormones play an important role in every woman's life. They shape our bodies as well as some of the most important events we experience, from pregnancy and childbirth to the menopause.

## Changes in the Breast Associated with Ageing

As a woman ages, her breasts normally change in certain ways.

As a woman gets beyond menopause, her breasts begin to change. These changes are associated with lower levels of the female hormone estrogen and may include:

- a loss of fullness in the breasts
- sagging and flattening of the breasts
- a decrease in the size of the nipples
- a reduction in the ability of the nipples to respond to stimulation
- replacement of milk-producing breast glands with fat

Since the sagging of the breasts is a normal part of aging, there are no exercises that can prevent the change. Exercise that results in weight loss will reduce breast size, and weight gain will cause breast enlargement.

Other changes in the breast may be abnormal. The risk of breast cancer rises with age. When caught early, breast cancer often responds to treatment. A woman should do a breast self-examination once a month. Self-exams help a woman learn how her breasts normally feel. Any lumps or changes should be reported to a healthcare provider.

Chapter 6
# Estrogen and the Risk of Breast Cancer

## The Role of Estrogen[71]

Estrogen is a hormone that is a chemical messenger in the body. It is important for normal sexual development and for the normal functioning of the female organs needed for childbearing such as the ovaries and uterus. Estrogen helps control a woman's menstrual cycle. It is important for the normal development of the breast. It also helps maintain healthy bones and the heart. All of these are tissues that estrogen can influence. During the childbearing years from puberty to menopause, organs called the ovaries produce estrogen. After menopause, when the ovaries no longer make estrogen, body fat is the primary source for estrogen made by the body.

## Estrogen and the risk of breast cancer

The effect of ovarian hormones, such as estrogen, on breast cancer risk was first shown over 100 years ago when researchers found that removing the ovaries of women with breast cancer improved their chances of survival. Women who experience menarche at an early age, that is before 12 years, or menopause after 55 years of age (when a woman's periods end), have a higher risk of breast cancer. This leads to a woman having more number of menstrual cycles, and hence the length of exposure to estrogen during her lifetime increases which in turn affects her risk for breast cancer.

## How does estrogen work?

**As a messenger:** During each menstrual cycle, estrogen together with other ovarian hormones signals cells in the breast to divide and multiply. Estrogen also signals the cells of the uterus to divide. Other hormones signal the ovaries to make estrogen, and then the ovaries secrete estrogen into the bloodstream. Estrogen travels through the blood, but only the cells in estrogen target tissues, like the breast and uterus, can recognize and use estrogen because they have estrogen receptors.

**As a key in a lock:** Estrogen has a shape that allows it to fit into an estrogen receptor in the same way a key fits into a 'lock.' The estrogen and the estrogen receptor bind to form a unit which binds to specific regulatory sites on the cell's DNA. These specialized genes instruct the cell to make proteins that signal the cell to carry out important activities. Some of these signaling proteins can tell the cell to divide.

**As different versions of the same key:** Estrogen is present in the body in different forms. The estrogen receptor can bind with these different forms of estrogen—much like when one lock can be opened by more than one key. Some forms of estrogen are stronger than others. Stronger forms are more likely to initiate cell division than weaker forms. In addition, some forms of estrogen stay in the body longer than others.

## How can estrogen affect the development of breast cancer?

**Cell division and the cancer process:** One characteristic of a cancer cell is that it multiplies out of control. The progression from a normal cell to a cancer cell is a multistep process that includes the build-up of damage to the DNA in key genes that control cell division.

Damage to a gene in DNA is called a mutation. This damage may happen in several different ways. Rarely, a child may inherit a mutated gene from a parent. For example, the breast cancer genes BRCA1 and BRCA2 may have mutations that parents can pass on to children. More commonly, a chemical or radiation that damages the

DNA may cause mutations. Another cause of DNA damage is when a mutation arises by chance. The chance mutation is a result of the cell making a mistake in copying its DNA during cell division.

Since estrogen stimulates cell division, it can increase the chance of making a DNA copying error in a dividing breast cell. Estrogen can also have the effect of making a spontaneous or chemically-induced mutation permanent, since it influences the rate of cell division. Because mistakes in DNA become permanent if the cell divides and passes on the mutation, estrogen-stimulated cell division can increase the chance of making a mutation permanent.

**The critical periods of breast growth and development:** The breast is unique because unlike other organs (such as the liver) that are fully formed at birth, the breast in the newborn girl consists of only a few tiny ducts.

Stimulating the development of the breast ducts is an important normal function of estrogen. However, immature breast cells are particularly sensitive to the effects of cancer-causing agents, called carcinogens. Animal studies have shown that rapidly dividing, immature cells of the developing breast are more likely to bind carcinogens. The immature stem cells are also less efficient at repairing damage to DNA caused by carcinogens. Stages when immature breast cells are particularly vulnerable to damage by carcinogens include 0-4 years of age and from puberty to a woman's first full term pregnancy. During pregnancy, breast cells undergo changes that protect them against damage caused by carcinogens.

**Effects on other hormones that stimulate cell division:** Estrogen can indirectly stimulate cell division by instructing a target cell to make receptors for other hormones that stimulate breast cells to divide. For instance, estrogen affects the receptor levels of a female hormone called progesterone. In the breast, progesterone also acts as a chemical messenger that tells breast cells to divide. It may affect how the cell responds to 'local' hormones called growth factors which also play a role in breast cell division. So, by affecting the level of other hormone receptors or growth factors, estrogen can indirectly stimulate cell division in the breast.

**Support of the growth of estrogen responsive tumors:** About one to two-thirds of all breast tumors have estrogen receptors and depend on estrogen for growth. That is why doctors often prescribe the anti-estrogen Tamoxifen for women who have estrogen-receptor positive breast tumors. Anti-estrogens can block the binding of estrogen to its receptor, and thereby prevent estrogen from delivering its message to the breast tumor cells to divide and multiply. Also, women who have a first full-term pregnancy late in life may be at increased risk for developing breast cancer. This is because by the time they get pregnant estrogen-responsive breast tumor cells may have formed, and the high levels of estrogen secreted during pregnancy may promote growth of the estrogen-responsive breast tumor cells.

## What influences estrogen level in the body?

A variety of different factors that may enhance or reduce a woman's exposure to estrogen. These include lifestyle factors like diet, body fat, alcohol consumption, hormone replacement therapy, birth control, and exercise. Whether exposure to chemicals that act like estrogen in a woman's body and to chemicals that disrupt the way estrogen works in a woman's body due to environmental exposure is being studied further.

## Breast Lumps may Appear at all Ages:[72, 73]

- Infants may have breast lumps related to estrogen from the mother. The lump generally goes away on its own as the estrogen clears from the baby's body. It can happen to boys and girls.
- Young girls often develop 'breast buds' that appear just before the beginning of puberty. These bumps may be tender. They are common around age 9, but may happen as early as age 6.
- Teenage boys may develop breast enlargement and lumps because of hormonal changes in mid-puberty. Although this may distress the teen, the lumps or enlargement generally go away on their own over a period of months.
- Breast lumps in an adult woman raises concern for breast cancer, even though most lumps turn out to be not cancerous.

## Common causes

Lumps in a woman are often caused by fibrocystic changes, fibro adenomas, and cysts.

Fibrocystic changes can occur in either or both breasts. These changes occur in many women (especially during the reproductive years) and are considered a normal variation of breast tissue. Having fibrocystic breasts does not increase your risk for breast cancer. It does, however, make it more difficult to interpret lumps that you or your doctor find on exam. Many women feel tenderness in addition to the lumps and bumps associated with fibrocystic breasts.

Fibro adenomas are non-cancerous lumps that feel rubbery and are easily moveable within the breast tissue. Like fibrocystic changes, they occur most often during the reproductive years. Usually, they are not tender and, except in rare cases, do not become cancerous later. A doctor may feel fairly certain from an exam that a particular lump is a fibro adenoma. The only way to be sure, however, is to remove or biopsy them.

Cysts are fluid-filled sacs that often feel like soft grapes. These can sometimes be tender, especially just before your menstrual period. Cysts may be drained in the doctor's office. If the fluid removed is clear or greenish, and the lump disappears completely after it is drained, no further treatment is needed. If the fluid is bloody, it is sent to the lab to look for cancer cells. If the lump doesn't disappear, or recurs, it is usually removed surgically.

## Other causes of breast lumps include

- Milk cysts (sacs filled with milk) and infections (mastitis), which may turn into an abscess. These typically occur if you are breastfeeding or have recently given birth.
- Breast cancer, detectable by mammogram or ultrasound, then a biopsy. Men can also get breast cancer.
- Injury—sometimes if your breast is badly bruised, there will be a collection of blood that feels like a lump. These tend to resolve on their own in a matter of days or weeks. If not, the blood may have to be drained by your doctor.

- Lipoma—a collection of fatty tissue.
- Intraductal papilloma—a small growth inside a milk duct of the breast. Often occurs near the areola, the coloured part of the breast surrounding the nipple, in women between the ages of 35 and 55. It is harmless and frequently cannot be felt. In some cases the only symptom is a watery, pink discharge from the nipple. Since a watery or bloody discharge can be seen in cases of breast cancer, this must be evaluated by your doctor.

## The spread of breast cancer

1. **Local spread:** The tumor increases in size and spreads to other portions of the breast. It tends to involve the skin, the pectoral muscles and even the chest wall.
2. **Lymphatic spread:** Occurs primarily to the axillary (armpit) lymph nodes and to the internal mammary (chest) chain of lymph nodes. The involvement of the nodes indicates the spread of the cancer. Involvement of supraclavicular (above collar bone) nodes and contralateral nodes (on the other side) suggests that the disease is in advanced stage.
3. **Spread by blood stream:** Through blood, spread of cancer can occur to the bones such as vertebrae (spine), femur, ribs and skull and also to distant organs of the body.

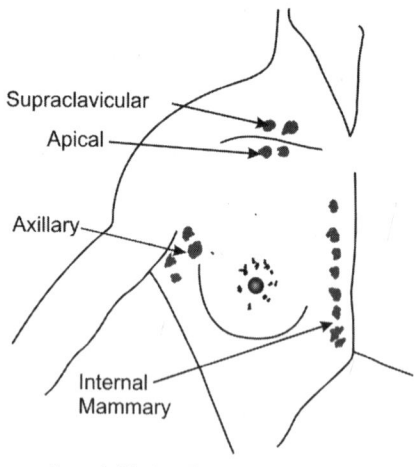

Lymph Nodes Draining the Breast

Chapter 7

# Types of Breast Cancer

## Ductal Carcinoma in Situ[74, 75, 76]

Ductal cancer in situ (DCIS), means that cells inside some of the ducts of your breast have started to turn into cancer cells. As these cells are all inside the ducts, there is very little chance that any of the cells have spread to the lymph nodes or elsewhere in the body. In the staging system that doctors use to classify cancer, DCIS is known as Stage 0. And it is sometimes called 'pre-cancer.' It is also referred to as TIS, which means that the cancer is non-invasive. TIS stands for 'tumor in situ' or 'in the same place.' DCIS hasn't started to break through normal tissue, which means it's not life-threatening like cancer. However, DCIS still requires careful medical treatment. More and more DCIS are being picked up by mammograms done for screening of breast cancer.

## DCIS grade

There are now ways of classifying DCIS into high grade (more aggressive) and low grade (less aggressive). There is also an intermediate grade that is in between high grade and low grade. Doctors think that the high grade is more likely to come back. So women with high grade should probably have radiotherapy after surgery. While women with low grade DCIS probably do not need further treatment.

## Treatment

Most centers remove only the area of DCIS, with a border of healthy tissue around it. This is called wide local excision or conservative surgery. The DCIS cells are examined under a microscope, and if they are of high grade, radiation therapy is suggested to the rest of the breast tissue. This is to kill any abnormal cells left behind. You may be given tamoxifen (a type of hormone therapy) to try to reduce the risk of developing an invasive breast cancer in the future.

You may be advised to have a mastectomy if:

- The area of the DCIS in your breast is large
- There are several areas of DCIS in your breast
- You have small breasts and too much of the breast is affected by DCIS to make wide local excision possible

## Follow up

Whichever treatment you receive, you will have regular follow up appointments to make sure any recurrence of DCIS in the treated breast is picked up as quickly as possible. Screening with mammograms would be advised. If your DCIS does come back, your specialist will probably suggest a mastectomy.

# Lobular Carcinoma in Situ (LCIS)

It is a pre-cancerous growth that begins in the milk-producing glands (lobules). It does not penetrate through the wall of the lobules, and most researchers believe it does not usually become an invasive breast cancer. However, women who develop lobular carcinoma in situ have a higher future risk of developing invasive breast cancer in the same or opposite breast.

## Follow up

If you have been treated for a lobular carcinoma in situ, you will want to have a physical exam two or three times a year, in addition to an annual mammogram.

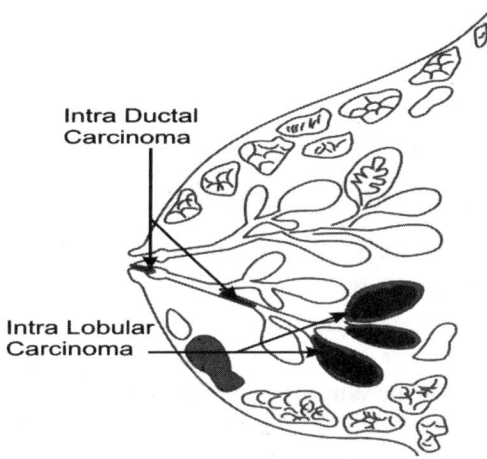

Location of Carcinomas

## Invasive Ductal Carcinoma

Invasive ductal carcinoma accounts for nearly 80% of breast cancers. Invasive means that it has 'invaded' or spread to the surrounding tissues. It is ductal because the cancer began in the milk ducts–which are the 'pipes' that bring milk from the lobules to the nipple.

It also begins in a milk duct, but unlike ductal carcinoma in situ, it invades the fatty tissue of the breast. This invasive carcinoma has the potential to spread to other parts of the body through the bloodstream or lymphatic system. It is important to detect and treat invasive ductal carcinoma before it has had time to spread to other organs.

- There are different types of invasive ductal breast cancer. These do not make much difference to you. They are treated the same way. But we have included them so that you know what the doctor means if you hear the terms used.

Most often, ductal carcinoma is described as being of no special type. You may see this written as NST or NOS (not otherwise specified).

## Treatment

For ductal breast cancer, you may have

- Surgery

- Radiotherapy
- Chemotherapy
- Hormone therapy

## Invasive Lobular Breast Cancer

Invasive lobular carcinoma, or ILC, accounts for about 10%–15% of all breast cancers. Invasive means that it has 'invaded' or spread to the surrounding tissues. It is lobular because the cancer began in the lobules–the glands that actually make milk. Carcinoma refers to any cancer that begins in the skin or other tissues that line or cover internal organs–such as breast tissues. This means that the cancer is growing in the cells that line the lobules of the breast. Invasive lobular cancer can develop in women of any age. But it is most common in women between 45 and 55 years of age. The outlook for invasive lobular breast cancer is much the same as for ductal breast cancer. It is more common for it to be diagnosed in both breasts at the same time. And if you have invasive lobular breast cancer diagnosed in one breast, there is a slightly higher risk than there is for ductal breast cancer of getting it in the other breast in the future.

### Symptoms and diagnosis

Invasive lobular breast cancer does not always show up as a firm lump. And it does not form the pattern on a mammogram called calcification. So it can be difficult to diagnose. Due to this, generally speaking, invasive lobular cancers may be larger than other types of breast cancer when they are diagnosed. You may have a thickened area of breast tissue instead of a definite lump.

Invasive lobular breast cancer can sometimes be found in more than one area within the breast. If this is the case, it may not be possible to remove just the area of the cancer. You may be asked to have a mastectomy. If at all possible, your breast surgeon will offer you the choice of local surgery or mastectomy.

## Treatment

- Surgery
- Chemotherapy
- Radiation therapy
- Hormonal therapy

## Inflammatory Breast Cancer

This is a rare type of breast cancer. Only about 1 or 2 breast cancers out of every 100 diagnosed (1 or 2%) are of this type. It is called 'inflammatory' because the breast becomes inflamed. The cancer cells block the smallest lymph channels in the breast. The lymph channels (or lymph ducts) are part of the lymphatic system. Their job is to drain excess tissue fluid away from the body tissues and organs.

## Symptoms

Because the lymph channels are blocked, the breast becomes

- Swollen
- Red
- Hot to the touch

The breast can also be painful in inflammatory breast cancer, but this is not always the case. Other possible symptoms include

- Ridges or thickening of the skin of the breast
- Pitted skin, like orange peel
- A lump in the breast
- A discharge from the nipple
- Inverted nipple—the nipple is pulled into the breast

Inflammatory breast cancer symptoms can come on quite suddenly. It is often confused with an infection of the breast (mastitis) because the symptoms are very similar. You may have been given a course of antibiotics at first, to see if that would clear the condition up. The same tests are used to diagnose inflammatory breast cancer as for any other type of breast cancer. In some cases, it is not possible to do a mammogram because the breast is swollen and painful.

## Treatment

The treatment for inflammatory breast cancer can be slightly different than for other types of breast cancer.

Usually, chemotherapy is the first treatment you have. This is called neo adjuvant chemotherapy. You have this first to help control the condition in the breast and reduce the swelling. The chemotherapy also travels throughout the body and so will attack any breast cancer cells that have broken away and spread outside the breast.

After chemotherapy, you are most likely to have surgery. Mastectomy is the commonest operation for inflammatory breast cancer - this means removing the whole breast. Or you may be able to have just the affected area removed. This will depend on

- The size of the cancer when you were diagnosed
- How the cancer has responded to the chemotherapy
- Where the tumor is in the breast

You may also have radiotherapy and hormone therapy after your surgery, to try to reduce the risk of the cancer coming back.

## Paget's Disease

Paget's disease is a rare disease that is associated with breast cancer. It is found in 1 or 2 out of every 100 breast cancers (1 to 2%).

Paget's disease starts in the nipple or in the area of darker skin surrounding it (the areola). It usually first appears as a red, scaly rash of the skin over the nipple and areola. It can be itchy. If it isn't treated, or if you scratch it, it can bleed, ulcerate and may scab over. It may be mistaken for eczema, both by women and their doctors. It has a reputation for late diagnosis, probably because it is often first treated as eczema, before any cancer investigations are done.

Paget's disease is diagnosed from a biopsy. Your breast surgeon will take a sample of the affected skin tissue (a biopsy) from the nipple and send it to be examined under a microscope. If Paget's disease is diagnosed, you will then have a mammogram. In many cases, Paget's disease is a sign that there is a breast cancer in the breast tissues behind the nipple. About half the women diagnosed with Paget's disease have a lump or mass behind the nipple. In 9 out of 10 cases, this is an invasive breast cancer.

About 4 out of 10 of the women with Paget's disease who do not have a lump also have an invasive breast cancer. But most just have carcinoma in situ. This means there are cancer cells in the biopsy, but that they are contained. This is not an invasive breast cancer and so there is no chance that the cancer cells have spread. If left untreated, a carcinoma in situ can go on to develop into an invasive cancer.

How is it treated? Generally, the treatment for Paget's disease is much the same as for any other breast cancer. You will have surgery to have either the whole breast removed or just the affected area removed. Further treatment depends on whether your results show that you have an invasive breast cancer, or not.

If you are found to have an invasive breast cancer, after surgery, you may have

- Radiotherapy
- Chemotherapy
- Hormone therapy

The exact choice of treatment will depend on the results of your surgery.

Mastectomy may be the only option if you have a large area affected by Paget's or if there is an area of invasive breast cancer behind the nipple. With a cancer is placed centrally in the breast, your surgeon may not be able to leave you with a satisfactory breast shape if you have surgery just to remove the cancer and surrounding tissue. You may get a better cosmetic result if you have the whole breast removed and then have breast reconstruction. For some women, it is possible to just have the area containing the cancer removed, together with a border of healthy tissue. This will be followed by a course of radiotherapy to the rest of the breast.

If your breast cancer cells are found to have estrogen receptors your doctor will probably suggest that you have treatment with 5 years of

tamoxifen (or other similar hormone treatment). This is to reduce the risk of
- The cancer coming back in the same breast
- Getting a new cancer in the other breast

Your doctor may suggest further treatment with chemotherapy if there is a significant risk that the cancer may come back. This could be because
- Cancer cells were found in your lymph nodes
- You had a large breast tumor
- Your cancer cells were high grade (grade 3)

Giving chemotherapy helps to lower the risk of the cancer coming back in the future.

## If there is no breast lump

Mastectomy is still the most commonly used treatment for Paget's disease where there is no invasive breast cancer. This is because the cells are abnormal and could develop into an invasive breast cancer if not treated. Your surgeon will remove some lymph nodes to check for signs of cancer. In 9 out of 10 cases, there is no sign of cancer in the lymph nodes. But it is best to make sure. In most cases, the surgery will be all the treatment you need.

If the affected area is not too large, you may just be able to have just the Paget's removed, along with a border of healthy tissue around it. Your doctor is likely to advise that you have radiotherapy after your surgery. Without it, there is quite a high risk that the Paget's will come back. Even with only local surgery, your surgeon will still want to remove some of your lymph nodes to check them.

## Recurrent and Metastatic Disease

If you've had breast cancer, the possibility of recurrence and spread of breast cancer stays with you.

Keep in mind that a recurrence of breast cancer or metastatic (advanced) disease is not without hope. Many women continue to live long, productive lives with breast cancer of this stage.

Chapter 8

# When and how to Perform Breast Self Examination (BSE)[77]

## Women who Menstruate

Women experience changes in their breast tissue every month due to changes in hormone levels that occur during the menstrual cycle (the span of time from the start of one period to the start of the next). These changes in the hormone levels cause the breasts to swell. The swelling decreases with the menstrual flow and the breasts return to their normal size. Due to this cycle, the best time to examine your breasts is about a week after start of your period that is when the breasts are least likely to be swollen or tender. For women who are lactating BSE can be performed after having given the feed so that breasts are emptied. Those who have either undergone surgery or have breast implants should also perform BSE.

## Women who do not Menstruate

For women who do not menstruate or who have irregular menstrual cycles can perform BSE on the same date each month.

## Lumpy Breasts

Fibrocystic disease is a common condition of the breast. It is neither cancerous nor does it increase the chances of suffering from a breast cancer. This condition most frequently results from changes in hormone levels that occur during menstruation or with peri-menopause and menopause. Having fibrocystic disease does not mean that one is more likely to develop a breast cancer. If your breasts are lumpy, performing BSE is more challenging. Becoming familiar with what is normal for you through regular BSE will help make detection of any new lumps or changes easier.[78]

## How to Recognize Breast Cancer (Symptoms)[79]

i. Lump or mass in the breast / armpit.
ii. Change in the shape and size of the breast.
iii. Nipple discharge (especially blood).
iv. Skin changes like dimpling, skin resembling that of an orange peel or retraction of the nipple.

## Screening of breast cancer

1. Breast Self Examination (BSE)
2. Clinical Breast Examination (CBE): By doctor or trained personnel
3. Mammography

| Age (Years) | BSE | CBE | Mammogram |
|---|---|---|---|
| 20 | Monthly | Nil | Nil |
| 20-39 | Monthly | Every 3 years | Nil |
| 40 and Over | Monthly | Yearly | Yearly |

# The techniques of Breast self examination

Remember the seven P's for a complete Breast Self Examination
1. Positions
2. Perimeter
3. Palpation
4. Pressure
5. Pattern
6. Practice with feed back
7. Plan of Action

## 1. Positions

Remove the entire clothes waist upwards. While standing in front of the mirror in which you can see this exposed area, visually inspect your breasts looking for changes in contour and shape, color and texture of the skin and nipple and evidence of discharge from the nipples moving from side to side.

The inspection should be done in 4 positions while standing in front of the mirror:

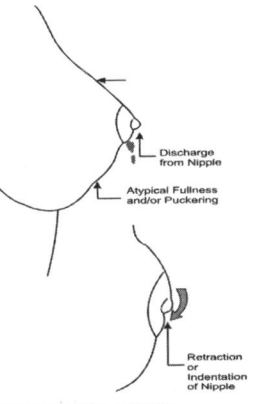

Visual Inspection of Breast

(i) Arms relaxed at sides and inspect from moving slowly from one side to the other.

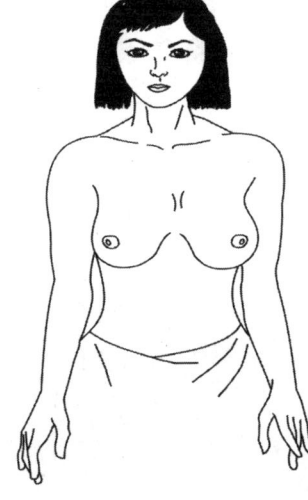

(ii) Arms raised above the head: raise your arms over your head and look at your breasts as you turn slowly from side to side.

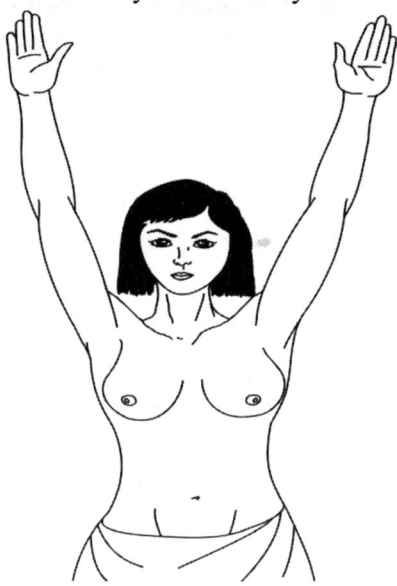

(iii) Hands on hips: press your hands on the hips and push your shoulders forwards and inspect from moving slowly from one side to the other.

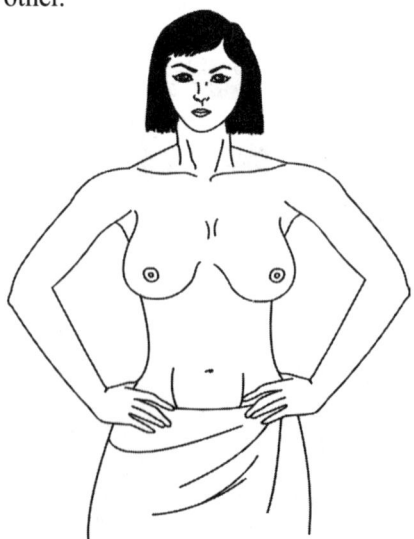

When and how to Perform Breast Self Examination(BSE)　　　　　63

(iv) Bending forwards and inspect from moving slowly from one side to the other.

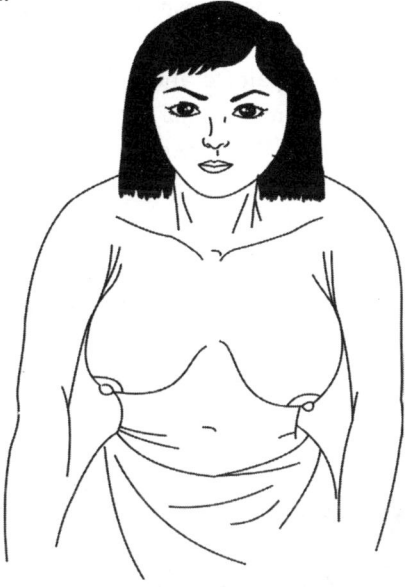

## 2. Perimeter

The examination area is bounded by a line which extends down from middle of the armpit to just beneath the breast, continues across along the underside of the breast to the middle of the breast bone then up to and along the collar bone and back to the middle of the armpit. Most of the breast cancers occur in the upper-outer area of the breast (shaded area in the diagram)

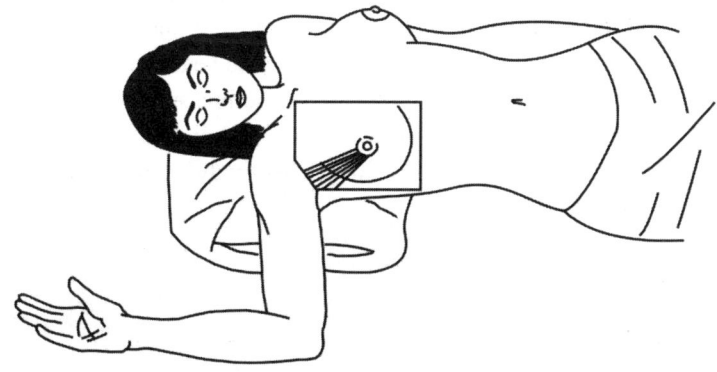

## 3. Palpation

(i) **Lying down:** It is the best position for manual examination. Two palpation positions are employed i) flat and ii) side lying. Use your left hand to palpate your right breast, while holding your right arm at right angle to the rib cage, with the elbow bent. Repeat the procedure on the other side. Some women prefer using BSE sensitivity pads which are now available in the market but their use is not advocated by any authority.

    a. **Flat position:** Lie flat on your back with either a pillow or folded towel under the shoulder of the breast to be examined. This enables the breast tissue to spread evenly so that the whole of the breast can be palpated without missing out any lumps.

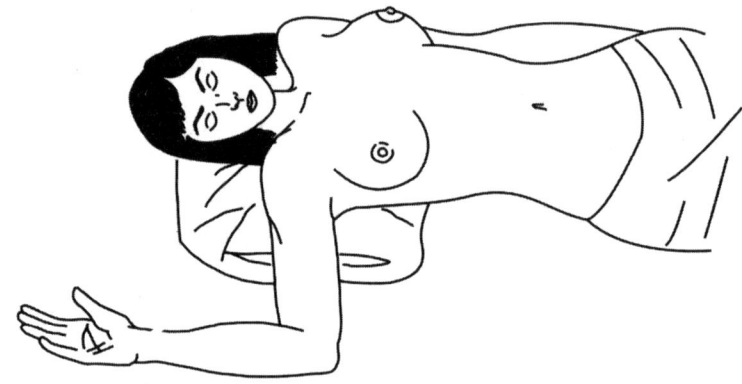

    b. **Side-lying position:** This position is for large breasted women. Lie on the opposite side of the breast to be examined. Rotate the shoulder on the same side of the breast to be examined with back to the flat surface. The side-lying position enables large breasted women to most effectively examine the outer portion of the breast.

# When and how to Perform Breast Self Examination(BSE)

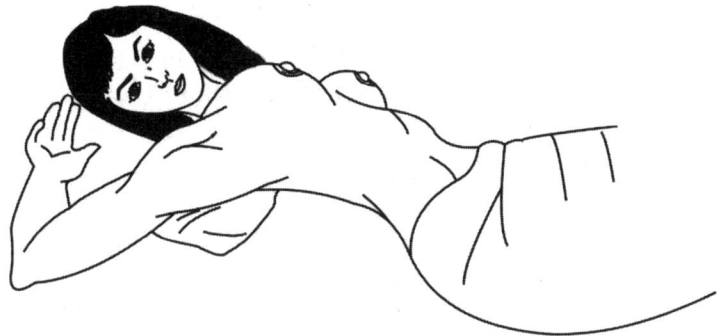

(ii) **Standing:** While standing in a shower, with a soapy hand that will help your fingers move smoothly, place your right hand behind your head and with your left hand check the entire right breast and chest area using three methods described below (vertical strip, wedge and circular massage). Then repeat the same procedure with your left hand behind your head.

## Palpation with the pads of the fingers

Use the pads of 3 fingers to examine every inch of your tissue. Pads of finger are most sensitive to touch than the tips and hence more likely to feel a lump. Move your fingers in circles about the size of a coin.

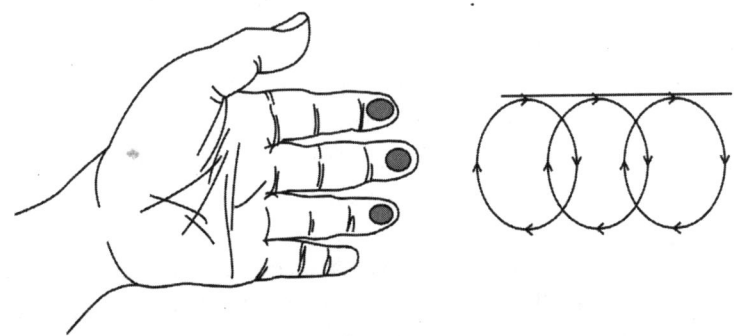

## 4. Pressure

Use varying levels of pressure for each palpation, from light to deep to examine the full thickness of your breast tissue. Using pressure will not injure the breast.

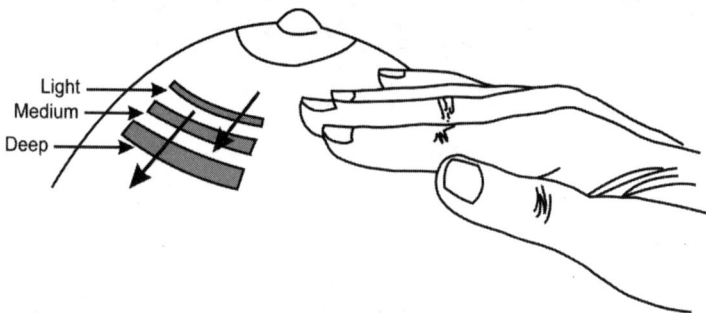

**Light:** move the skin without moving the tissue underneath

**Medium:** midway into the tissue

**Deep:** down to the ribs, 'on the verge of pain'

**Remember:** 3fingers, 3circles, 3pressures

## 5. Pattern of search during BSE

Use one of the following methods to examine all of the breast and armpit. Palpate carefully beneath the nipple. Any incision should be carefully examined from end to end. Women who have had any breast surgery should still examine the entire area and the incision.

(i) **Vertical strip:**[80] The National Cancer Institute developed the vertical or linear method of breast self examination. This method is now recommended by the American Cancer Society. Recent research suggests this up and down pattern of BSE is more thoroughly followed by many women. Start in the middle of the armpit, move downward to the lower boundary of breast. Move a finger's width toward the middle and continue palpating upward till you reach the collarbone. Continue like this until you have covered all the breast tissue. Make at least 6 strips before the nipple and four strips after the nipple. You may need between 10 and 16 strips.

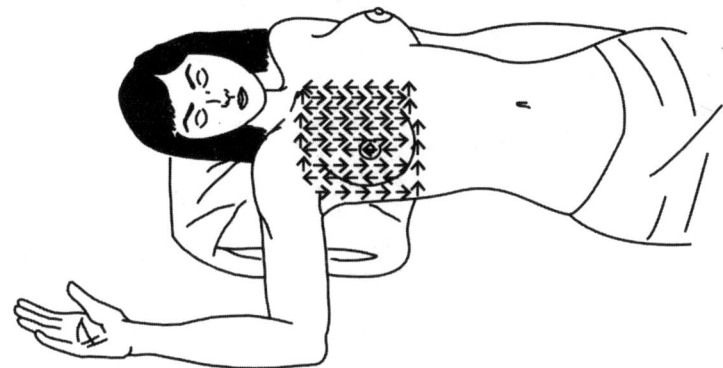

(ii) **Wedge:** Imagine your breast divided like spokes of a wheel with the nipple in the center. Examine each segment, moving from the outer boundary toward the nipple. Slide fingers back to the boundary, move over a finger's width and repeat this procedure until you have covered all breast tissue. You may need between 10 and 18 segments.

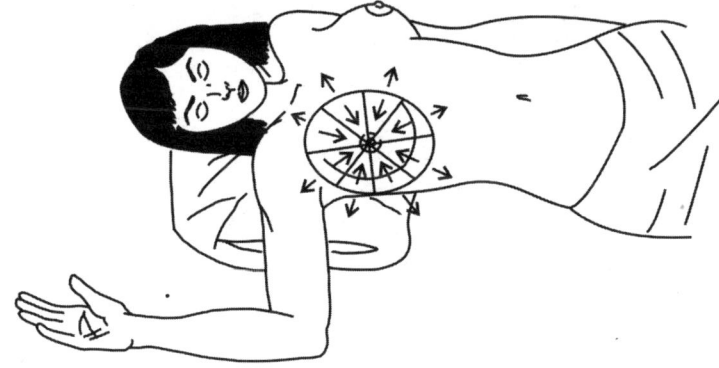

(iii) **Circle:** Imagine your breast as the face of a clock. Start at 12 o'clock and palpate along the boundary of each circle until you return to the starting point. Then move down a finger's width and continue palpating in ever-smaller circles until you reach the nipple. Depending on the size of your breast, you may need 8 to 10 circles.

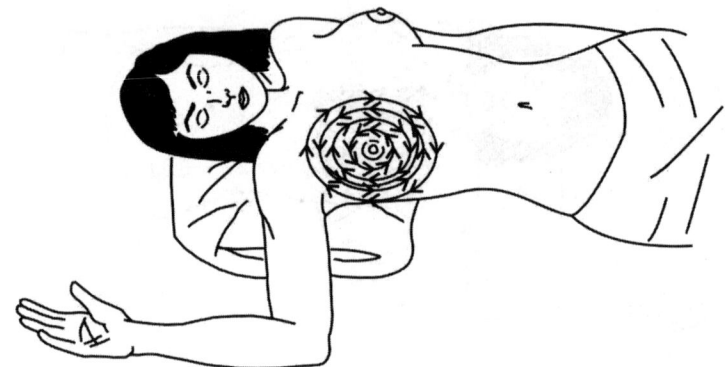

(iv) **Check for nipple discharge:** In many females there might be spontaneous discharge from one of the nipples especially that of blood and may indicate cancer. In many normal women there may be a clear or milky discharge.

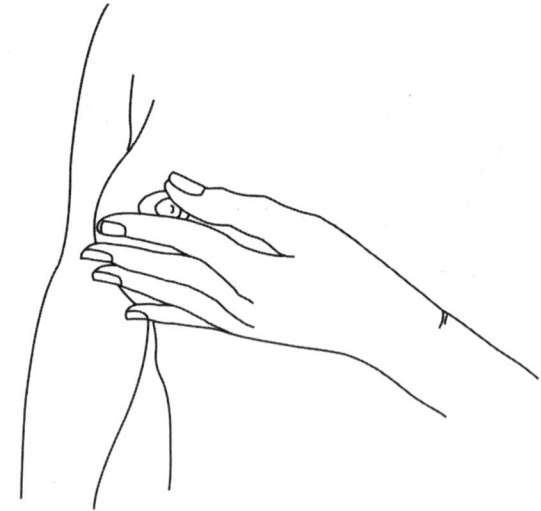

(v) **Armpit examination:** Examine the breast tissue that extends into your armpit while your arm is relaxed at your side.

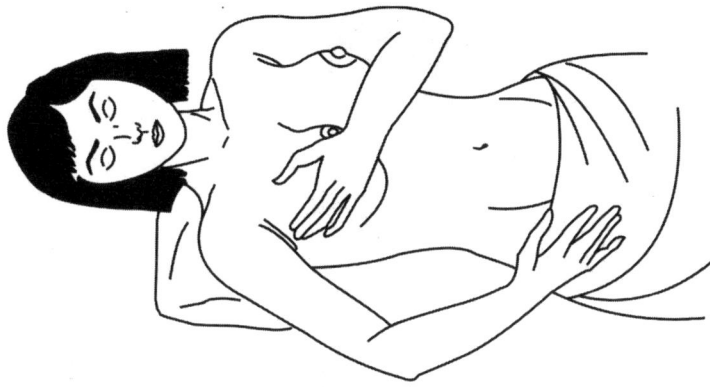

## What to feel for

Women should feel their breasts monthly so that they become familiar with what is normal for them. Many women have a normal thickening or ridge of firm tissue under the lower curve of the breast, at its attachment to the chest wall. Also the large milk ducts can be felt as a ring of bumps, at the outer edge of the areola. In very slender women, the bony prominences of the chest wall may be mistaken for chest tumors, as may be enlarged milk glands or benign cysts. All such thickenings should be palpated carefully during monthly BSE in order to distinguish stable, normal conditions from potentially dangerous changes. If any abnormal finding is there in one breast examine the same site on the other breast. Any lump or other change found in one breast only (especially in the upper outer quadrant) is more likely to be serious than a change, which has a mirror image in the other breast. In case of any doubt or change, do not panic, as most of these lumps are benign and contact your physician immediately.

## Record your observations

Date.... Month...... Year.......

Any change in the size, shape, colour, skin changes......

Any discharge.....

Any lump felt.....

Any increase in the size of a previous lump......

Any new lump felt.....

Action taken..........

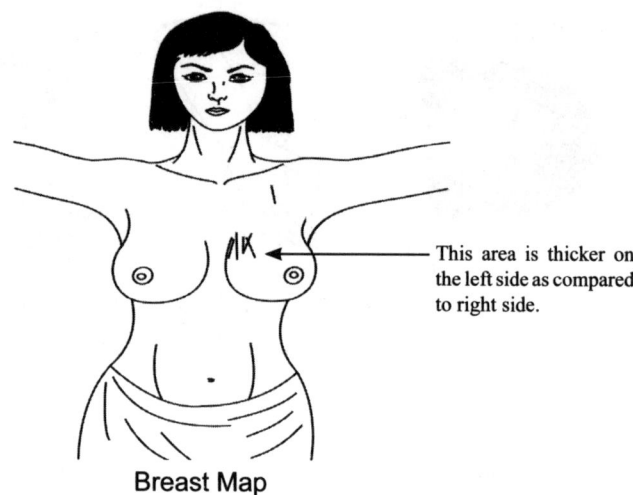

Breast Map

Maintain a note book and record your observations monthly.

## 6. Practice with feedback

It is important that you do Breast Self Examination while your instructor watches, to make sure that you are doing it correctly. Practice your skills under supervision until you feel comfortable and confident.

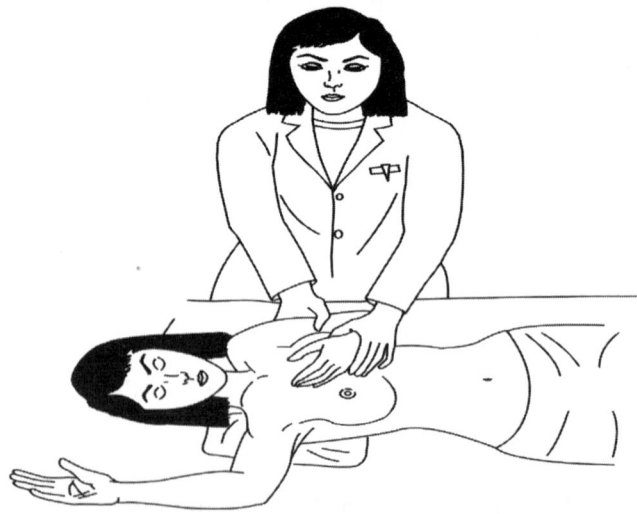

## 7. Plan of action

i. Report any changes to your doctor as soon as possible.
ii. Schedule your clinical breast examination and mammogram as appropriate.

Chapter 9

# How to Diagnose Breast Cancer

Breast self examination should be performed on regular basis by all women along with that a thorough clinical examination by your physician can reveal a lump at an early stage. However there are certain investigations which help in making a diagnosis.

## Mammograms[78,81,82,83]

An X- ray of the breast (mammogram) is the best tool available for early diagnosis even before symptoms appear. X-ray is taken after placing the breast in direct contact with an ultra sensitive film. Mammograms can often detect a breast lump and can also show small deposits of calcium in the breast. Although most calcium deposits are benign, a cluster of very tiny specks of calcium (called micro calcifications) may be an early sign of cancer. In young women in whom breasts are denser and more fibrous, a small percentage of breast cancers may not be visible on a mammogram, which otherwise may or may not be palpable by BSE or CBE.

## Ultrasonography

Using high frequency sound waves, ultrasonography can often show whether a lump is a fluid filled cyst (not cancer) or a solid mass (which may or may not be cancer). It is particularly useful in young women with dense breasts in whom mammograms are difficult to interpret. It can also be used to localize impalpable breast lumps.

## Fine needle aspiration cytology (FNAC)

A thin needle is put into the lump/mass and a tiny amount of fluid and or cells are removed from the breast lump and then smeared on to a slide to be checked by a pathologist. It is the least invasive technique of obtaining cells for diagnosis. False negatives do occur and invasive cancer cannot be distinguished from in situ disease. Ultrasound guided FNAC is a better technique, as it is more likely to get cells from the lump.

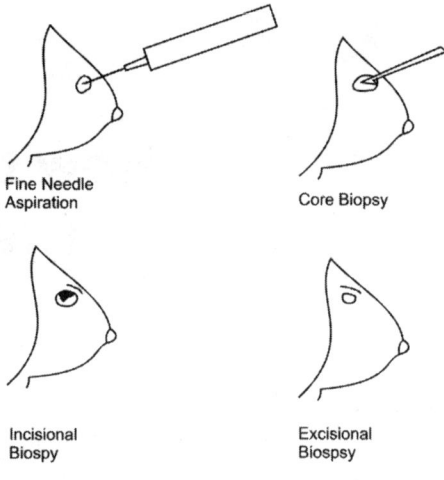

## Needle biopsy

Using a fine needle such as Trucut or Corecut biopsy device under local anesthesia tissue can be removed from the lump or an area that looks suspicious on the mammogram but cannot be felt. Tissue removed in a needle biopsy goes to a lab to be checked by a pathologist for cancer cells. Invasive cancer can be distinguished from in situ disease with needle biopsy.

## Surgical biopsy

In an incision biopsy, the surgeon cuts out a portion of a lump or suspicious area. In an excision biopsy, the surgeon removes all of the lump or suspicious area and an area of healthy tissue around the edge of the lump. A pathologist then examines the tissue under a microscope to check for cancer cells. A biopsy should not be performed before mammography as it may interfere with the interpretation of the results.

- Triple assessment consisting of clinical examination, Mammography and FNAC help in making the diagnosis of breast cancer.

- BSE only helps in finding a lump in it's early stage of development.

## Staging of Cancer

| Stage | Tumor | Node | Metastasis |
|---|---|---|---|
| Stage 0 | In situ | No spread | |
| Stage I | Up to 2 cms | No spread | |
| Stage II | <2cms | Has spread to axillary nodes | |
| | 2-5cms | May or may not have spread to axillary nodes | |
| | >5cms | No spread | |
| Stage III | Any size | Has spread to axillary nodes so that nodes become attached | |
| | >5 cms | Has spread to axillary nodes | |
| | Any size but cells have spread to skin or chest wall | May or may not have spread to the axillary lymph nodes | |
| | Any size | Has spread to the nodes along the breast bone or above/below collarbone | |
| Stage IV | Any size | May or may not have spread to axillary lymph nodes | Has spread to other organs of the body or the skin and nodes above the collar bone. |

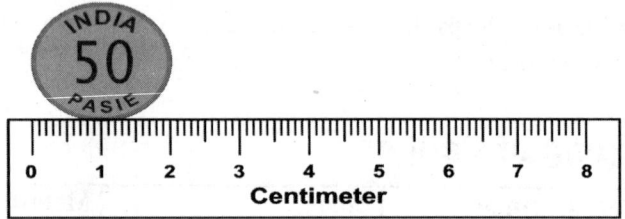

Size: 2 cms

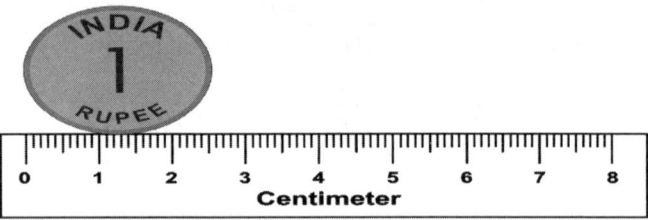

Size: 2.5 cms

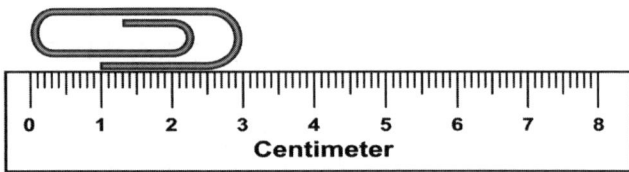

Size: 3cms

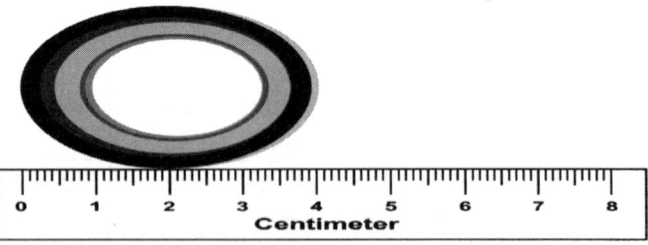

Size: 4 cms

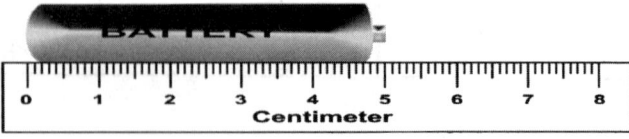

Size: 5 cms

## Chapter 10
# Pregnancy and Breast Cancer

Breast cancer is the most frequently seen cancer in pregnancy and lactation, but the incidence is low, the disease being seen in approximately 0.03% of pregnancies. Overall only 1 to 2% of the breast cancers are diagnosed during pregnancy or lactation.[84] Breast cancer is not very common during pregnancy, but as more women choose to have children later in life, it is expected to become more common in the future (because the risk of breast cancer increases with age). Pregnancy associated breast carcinoma (PABC) is defined as that being diagnosed during pregnancy, or within one year thereafter. Approximately 2-3% of all breast cancers coincide with pregnancy or lactation and this tumor affects only one to four out of 10,000 pregnant women, and is thus a rare occurrence.[85, 86, 87] Multiple studies have documented a delay in diagnosis in breast cancer during pregnancy. Generally, 40% to 50% of non pregnant young women with breast cancer present with disease metastatic to axillary lymph nodes. In contrast, several recent studies have documented lymph node metastasis in 56% to 89% of pregnant women with breast cancer. It appears that pregnancy and breast cancer are merely coincidental and that pregnancy or lactation does not directly contribute to the development or accelerated progression of breast cancer.[88] Pregnancy causes a number of hormonal changes in the body, one of which is an interruption of the normal menstrual cycle hormone levels. Because of this, women who have had a child or children at an earlier age may have a slightly lower risk of breast cancer. Women who have had no children or who had their first child after age 30 have a slightly higher breast cancer risk.

Some studies have suggested that breastfeeding may slightly lower breast cancer risk, especially if breastfeeding is continued for 1 ½ to 2 years or if several children are breastfed. The reason for this may be that both pregnancy and breastfeeding reduce a woman's total number of lifetime menstrual cycles. Not all studies, however, have found this impact on breast cancer risk, so more research is needed to answer this question more clearly. When breast cancer occurs during pregnancy, it is often diagnosed at a later stage than when diagnosed in women who are not pregnant. This is because during pregnancy, hormone changes cause the breasts to enlarge and become more glandular. This can make it harder for you or your doctor to find a lump in your breasts. Mammograms are also harder for doctors to read during pregnancy because of the increased density of the breasts. Normal changes in pregnancy make the evaluation of the breast difficult. Serial examinations are critical. The majority of breast lesions encountered during pregnancy are benign. The mortality of breast cancer during pregnancy is related to a delay in diagnosis.

Unfortunately, delay in diagnosis is common, and 70% to 89% of patients with operable cancer have positive axillary lymph nodes. Late stage appears to be the only reason for the generally worse prognosis in these patients, as stage for stage; they have a course similar to that of no pregnant patients.

## A Breast Cancer Diagnosis during Pregnancy[89, 90, 91]

The treatment of breast cancer during pregnancy should not be delayed unless a woman is within 2 to 3 weeks from her delivery date. Radiation, chemotherapy, and drug therapy are not typically given during pregnancy because they can potentially harm the fetus. However, recent studies show that women who receive chemotherapy during the second or third trimesters of pregnancy (after the first three months) still have good chances of having healthy babies. In more than one study, women who received chemotherapy during the second or third trimesters of pregnancy had live births and only a few had complications from the chemotherapy, such as early labor and low birth weight. However, the long-term effects of exposure to chemotherapy drugs during pregnancy are less well-studied and should be discussed in detail with treating physicians.

Surgery is commonly performed during pregnancy for a variety of conditions, and if proper care is taken during anesthesia and after surgery, generally no harm comes to the fetus. Typically, a mastectomy is recommended if breast cancer is diagnosed during the first or second trimester of pregnancy (the first six months). Mastectomy involves surgically removing the entire breast and often some or all of the axillary (underarm) lymph nodes. Mastectomy often prevents the need for radiation treatment. Chemotherapy or drug therapy is typically delayed until later in the pregnancy or after delivery, although the risks and benefits must be carefully weighted.

If breast cancer is diagnosed during the third trimester of pregnancy (the final three months), either mastectomy or breast-conserving therapy (i.e., lumpectomy) with lymph node removal may be performed as needed. Lumpectomy involves only removing the cancerous tumor and a surrounding margin of normal breast tissue. Radiation, chemotherapy, or drug therapy is usually delayed until after childbirth. Women who receive chemotherapy or other drug therapies after childbirth should not breast-feed because the drugs could be passed through the breast milk. Breast reconstruction is not typically performed until after childbirth and lactation, when the breasts return to their normal size and milk production has ceased completely

## Evaluating a Breast Abnormality during Lactation (Breast-Feeding)

If a worrisome breast lump or abnormality is found after birth when a woman is breast-feeding, diagnostic mammography and/or other breast imaging exams should not be delayed. Mammography is considered safe and can be accurate for women who are breast-feeding when performed with care. Some suggest that the breast should be completely emptied of milk immediately before the mammogram, either via nursing or breast pump. This decreases the density through which the x-rays must penetrate and helps improve image quality.

It is important to keep in mind that imaging tests are not foolproof and may not detect a mass even when it can be felt during a physical examination. Approximately 10% to 15% of breast masses are missed with mammography or ultrasound (sonography) in women who are not lactating, and this percentage can be as high as 25% in the denser, larger, lactating breast. For this reason, a breast abnormality detected during lactation will often need to be biopsied to determine whether it is cancerous or benign.

Fine needle aspiration (FNA) involves using a thin needle to sample fluid or cells from the breast. FNA is often used to identify or drain cysts (collections of fluid). Other biopsy methods, such as core needle biopsy or open surgical biopsy, can also be performed safely. However, these more invasive methods are usually reserved for cases when the diagnosis cannot be made by other, less invasive means. This is because milk fistulas (abnormal passages of milk) or collections of milk in the breast may result when a biopsy is performed on a lactating breast. Nevertheless, milk fistulas are rarely a problem and are more of an inconvenience compared with the more dangerous possibility of an undiagnosed breast cancer. If a biopsy is performed and a collection of milk does result, it can easily be drained by fine needle aspiration in the physician's office.

Diagnosis of breast cancer in pregnancy can be very difficult. New localized masses merit at least ultrasound examination and fine needle aspiration biopsy. For staging chest radiograph can be performed with abdominal and pelvic shielding.

## 1. Stage I or II

### First twelve weeks

Definitive therapy of breast cancer during this phase of pregnancy may endanger the fetus and therefore a therapeutic abortion is usually recommended. The treatment of the malignancy will then proceed as in the non-pregnant state. Patients who decline termination should be treated by a modified radical mastectomy. No adjuvant radiation therapy should be given during pregnancy. Chemotherapy with AC chemo has been given in this situation, but is avoided if possible, unless the risks of withholding chemo outweighed the risks to the fetus. Referral is recommended to assess the need for further treatment after the baby has been delivered.

### Twelve to twenty-eight weeks

During this interval the breast cancer can be adequately treated surgically without terminating pregnancy. Modified radical mastectomy is the treatment of choice. Adjuvant radiotherapy is contraindicated during pregnancy. The risk of recurrence should be estimated based on the pathology of the tumor. If the risk of relapse is high then adjuvant chemotherapy may be given.

### Twenty-eight weeks to term

Maturity of the fetus should be assessed. Consideration should be given to inducing labor as soon as obstetric advice indicates that the fetus is viable. Initial treatment by modified radical mastectomy is appropriate and as soon as the fetus has been delivered, the patient should receive additional treatment as for the non-pregnant state. Chemotherapy may be given during pregnancy but in most circumstances is delayed until after delivery.

### Lactation

When a carcinoma arises during lactation, lactation should be terminated and therapy appropriate for the treatment of the malignancy instituted.

## 2. Locally advanced or inflammatory breast cancer

Patients with advanced disease pose a special problem. In the early weeks of pregnancy consideration has to be given to termination of the pregnancy. If the patient is in the second trimester and is still hoping to deliver a viable child then chemotherapy with drugs least likely to harm the fetus, may be considered.

## Staging

Procedures used for staging of breast cancer should be modified to avoid radiation exposure to the fetus in pregnant women. Nuclear scans cause fetal radiation exposure. Timing of the exposure to radiation relative to the gestational age of the fetus may be more critical than the actual dose of radiation delivered. Radiation exposure during the first trimester can lead to congenital malformations, especially microcephaly. All radiological procedures, they should be used only when essential for making treatment decisions. For the diagnosis of bone metastases, a bone scan is preferable to a skeletal series because the bone scan delivers a smaller amount of radiation and is more sensitive. Evaluation of the liver can be performed with ultrasound, and brain metastases can be diagnosed with a magnetic resonance imaging (MRI) scan, both of which avoid fetal radiation exposure.

Overall survival of pregnant women with breast cancer may be worse than in non pregnant women at all stages. However, the decreased overall survival in this patient population may be due to primarily delayed diagnosis. Termination of pregnancy has not been shown to have any beneficial effect on breast cancer outcome and is not usually considered as a therapeutic option. However, termination of pregnancy may be considered based on the age of the fetus, if maternal treatment options such as chemotherapy and radiation therapy, are significantly limited by the continuation of the pregnancy.

## Treatment options

### Early stage disease (stages I and II)

Surgery is recommended as the primary treatment of breast cancer in pregnant women. Since radiation in therapeutic doses may expose the fetus to potentially harmful scatter radiation, modified radical mastectomy is the treatment of choice. Conservative surgery with postpartum radiation therapy has been used for breast preservation. An analysis has been performed which helps predict the risk of waiting to have radiation. If adjuvant chemotherapy is necessary, it should not be given during the first trimester to avoid the risk of teratogenicity. Chemotherapy given after the first trimester is generally not associated with a high risk of fetal malformation, but may be associated with premature labor and fetal wastage. If considered necessary, chemotherapy may be given after the first trimester. Data on the immediate and long-term effects of chemotherapy on the fetus are limited.

Studies using adjuvant hormonal therapy alone or in combination with chemotherapy for breast cancer in pregnant women are also limited. Therefore, no conclusion has been reached regarding these options. Radiation therapy, if indicated, should be withheld until delivery since it may be harmful to the fetus at any stage of development.

## Later stage disease (stages III and IV)

First-trimester radiation therapy should be avoided. Chemotherapy may be given after the first trimester as discussed above. As the mother may have a limited life span (most studies show a 5-year survival rate of 10% in pregnant patients with stages III and IV disease), and there is a risk of fetal damage with treatment during the first trimester, issues regarding continuation of the pregnancy should be discussed with the patient and her family. Therapeutic abortion does not improve prognosis.

## Fetal consequences of maternal breast cancer

No damaging effects on the fetus from maternal breast cancer have been demonstrated, and there are no reported cases of maternal-fetal transfer of breast cancer cells. The most common presentation of a malignant tumor is a painless lump, usually discovered by the patient.

Breast cancer during pregnancy involves a host of psychosocial, ethical, religious, and legal considerations; and historically has placed the welfare of the mother in conflict with that of the fetus. Although the diagnosis of breast cancer during pregnancy may be only a biological coincidence, the emotional impact of this coincidence can be devastating on both patient and family. Informed medical care and compassionate support are both essential for women who simultaneously must confront the diametrically opposed implications and expectations of a life-giving and a life-threatening process. Other special considerations with pregnancy-associated breast cancer include the timing of delivery, the potential for nursing and concerns for future fertility.

## Delayed diagnosis

Since breast cancer during pregnancy is not inherently a different disease from breast cancer in a young patient, the advanced stage of disease at presentation is more likely secondary to delay in diagnosis. There is an average reported delay of 5 to 15 months from the onset of symptoms. Physiologic changes during pregnancy modify the architecture of the breast considerably, and this may account for a significant portion of diagnostic delay. Due to the normal increase in secretion and release of ovarian placental estrogen and progestin during pregnancy, the breast enlarges, the ducts and lobules proliferate, and the breast prepares for active secretion. These changes dramatically alter the breast structure resulting in enlargement, firmness, and increased nodularity. The clinician examining the breast of a pregnant patient may mistake a dominant mass for the normal physiologic alterations of pregnancy. In addition, as the pregnancy progresses, these changes may become more pronounced, potentially obscuring a worrisome mass. As a result of these changes in the breast during pregnancy, delay in diagnosis occurs with disappointing frequency, possibly leading to poorer survival rates in pregnant as compared with non-pregnant women.

To detect breast cancer, pregnant and lactating women should practice regular judicious self-examination. A thorough and careful clinical breast examination of the pregnant females at the initial visit to the obstetrician before the breasts become enlarged and difficult to examine, is necessary, and should be continued thereafter. When a physician identifies a clinically suspicious, dominant mass-a-mass discrete and distinct from surrounding tissue-in a pregnant woman, proper referral and diagnosis are necessary.

There are 2 significant differences in diagnosing breast cancer in pregnant women compared to non-pregnant women. These involve the use of fine needle aspiration cytology (FNAC) and mammography. When a pregnant woman presents with a palpable, dominant breast mass, fine needle aspiration should be performed at the initial visit, as with a woman who is not pregnant. This technique is most useful in differentiating a cyst or galactocele from a solid lesion. If a solid mass is encountered, however, FNAC may be misleading. False-positive results have been reported and are believed to be due to hormonally related cellular atypia during pregnancy. Therefore, it is recommended that open biopsy be performed in a timely manner when a solid mass is identified during pregnancy. USG is a safe and accurate way to differentiate between solid and cystic lesions.

Mammography is widely employed by many physicians to aid in the evaluation of a suspicious breast mass. With proper shielding, mammograms should only be used to evaluate dominant masses and to locate occult carcinoma. A mammogram during pregnancy is not easy to read and has at least 25% false-negative rate because of the increased water content of the breast tissue and the loss of contrasting fatty tissue that usually defines a mass.

In the setting of pregnancy, open biopsy should be performed as FNAC and mammography during pregnancy are not adequate to make a diagnosis. Importantly, there is no evidence to suggest that a breast biopsy poses any significant anesthetic risk to either the fetus or the mother. The pathologist should be informed that the patient is pregnant in order to avoid a wrong diagnosis due to pregnancy related changes.

## Need for abortion

In the past, when it was thought that pregnancy itself detrimentally stimulated tumor growth, therapeutic abortion was an important element of breast cancer treatment. As it has become apparent that breast cancer during pregnancy is not inherently a different disease from breast cancer in a non-pregnant young woman, enthusiasm for abortion as a therapeutic maneuver has waned. Breast cancer in pregnancy is by itself not an indication for abortion. No damaging effects on the fetus from maternal breast cancer have been demonstrated, and there are no reported cases of maternal-fetal transfer of breast cancer cells.

Whether a woman proceeds with therapeutic abortion depends on the stage of pregnancy, the stage of disease, the desire for breast conservation, and the priorities of the individual patient. In an individual who insists on breast conservation therapy for a cancer discovered during the first trimester, therapeutic abortion may be preferable to exposing the fetus to ionizing radiation. Similarly, the dangers of teratogenesis from chemotherapy may convince a woman in her first trimester to terminate the pregnancy, allowing for therapy without hindrance. There is no evidence that termination of pregnancy improves the outlook for the patients or alter the natural history of breast cancer, but it does permit standard aggressive therapy in advanced disease. Hence therapeutic abortion should be performed in all women with advanced-stage disease and in whom a significant delay of this treatment would jeopardize maternal health.

However, since advanced-stage breast cancer is essentially incurable despite aggressive adjuvant therapy, the well-informed patient may wish to carry the pregnancy to term.

## Lactation during treatment

Suppression of lactation does not improve prognosis. However, if surgery is planned, lactation should be suppressed to decrease the size and blood supply of the breasts which also helps reduce the risk of infection in the breast, and can help avoid having breast milk collect in any previous biopsy incisions. It should also be suppressed if chemotherapy is to be given because many antineoplastics (specifically cyclophosphamide and methotrexate) given systemically may occur in high levels in breast milk and this would affect the nursing baby. In general, women receiving chemotherapy should not breast-feed.

## Breast biopsy during pregnancy and lactation

Biopsy can be performed safely using a cutting needle or open biopsy technique with suitable precautions to avoid hemorrhage (due to increased vascularity), hematoma formation, and milk fistula (during lactation).

## Breast changes during pregnancy and lactation (breast-feeding)

During pregnancy, increased levels of the hormones estrogen and progesterone stimulate a variety of breast changes. Typically, the breasts become tender and the nipples become sore a few weeks after conception. The Montgomery's gland surrounding the areola (the pigmented region around the nipple) becomes darker and more prominent, and the areola itself darkens.

One of the most common changes stimulated by the hormones of pregnancy is a rapid period of breast growth, especially during the first eight weeks of pregnancy. In fact, it is not uncommon for a woman's breasts to increase by one or two cup sizes during pregnancy and lactation. Later in the first trimester of pregnancy, levels of the two hormones responsible for milk production, prolactin and oxytocin, begin to increase. Prolactin is sometimes referred to as the 'mothering hormone' because some people believe it also causes a tranquilizing effect that makes women feel more maternal. The body begins producing prolactin approximately eight weeks after conception. As the pregnancy progresses, the levels of prolactin steadily increase, peaking when the woman gives birth. As the body produces more and more prolactin, high levels of estrogen and progesterone block some of the prolactin receptors and inhibit milk production until after the baby is born.

After birth, estrogen and progesterone levels decrease and the production of prolactin declines. The breasts will usually begin to produce milk three to five days after a woman has given birth. During these few days before milk is produced, the breasts secrete colostrum, a liquid substance that contains antibodies to help protect the infant against infections. Some physicians believe that colostrum also decreases an infant's chances of developing asthma and other allergies. Within a few days, the infant's need for high levels of the maternal antibodies in the colostrum decreases. At about the same time, the breasts begin to produce milk, which contains lower levels of antibodies that are passed on to the infant during breast-feeding. These antibodies are believed to decrease the infant's susceptibility to disease and infections in early life.

The other hormone responsible for milk production, oxytocin which triggers the delivery of milk that prolactin has produced. When an infant suckles at the mother's breast, milk is actively drawn out of the nipples by the suckling action and passively delivered to the infant by the contraction of small muscles surrounding the ducts in the breast. This process is commonly called the let-down reflex. The infant's suction signals the body to produce more milk (using prolactin) and deliver more milk (using oxytocin). A variety of other hormones that stimulate growth and development in the infant are also delivered in the breast milk including insulin thyroid, and cortisol.

A woman's body continues to produce milk until she stops breast-feeding or mechanically pumping breast milk. Even then, it may take several months for milk production to completely stop. The breasts usually return to their previous size, or slightly smaller, after breast-feeding is completed.

## Breast Health Guidelines during Pregnancy

A woman should continue practicing monthly breast self-exams during pregnancy at about seven to ten days after her normal period would have occurred. It is especially important that a clinical breast exam be performed by the physician or nurse during the first doctor's appointment of the pregnancy, before the breasts go through significant physiological changes. Some changes or lumps are more difficult to evaluate once the breasts have enlarged and have become more nodular. Clinical breast exams should continue on a monthly basis during pregnancy.

A main concern with breast cancer during pregnancy is a delay in the detection of a breast abnormality. The changes that occur during pregnancy may make cancers more difficult to diagnose and may result in a woman being diagnosed with breast cancer at a more advanced stage, when the chances of successful treatment and survival are lower. Vigilant monthly breast self-exams and clinical breast exams during pregnancy and lactation (breast-feeding) can help prevent the delayed diagnosis of breast cancer and enable optimal treatment.

Screening mammograms in asymptomatic women (women who have no symptoms of breast cancer) are not performed during pregnancy or lactation and may be performed at a later time. However, if a breast abnormality (such as a strange lump) is detected during pregnancy, a diagnostic mammogram or both/or ultrasound (sonogram) may be performed. A lead apron is usually placed over the woman's stomach/abdomen area during the mammogram to shield the developing fetus.

## Evaluating a breast abnormality during pregnancy

The hormonal changes during pregnancy and lactation (breast-feeding) may influence the growth of estrogen-sensitive tumors. Non-cancerous tumors are common during pregnancy and their growth may be stimulated by increased hormone levels. However, all breast lumps and abnormalities should be evaluated by a physician to distinguish between the more common benign changes and the potentially malignant (cancerous) ones.

## Non-cancerous conditions that are common during pregnancy include:

- Cysts (collections of fluid)
- Galactoceles (milk-filled cysts)
- Fibroadenomas (tumors; existing ones may enlarge during pregnancy)

It is fairly common for the nipples to discharge small amounts of milky, clear or sometimes bloody fluid during pregnancy and lactation. During pregnancy and lactation, breast tissue grows rapidly. Rapid tissue growth can lead to irritation of the breast ducts, causing nipple discharge. This discharge, whether blood or other fluid, is usually related to a non-cancerous condition, such as shedding of the cells lining the breast ducts or a papilloma (a benign wart-like growth). However, patients should consult their physicians if they experience nipple discharge to determine whether the discharge requires further examination.

If a breast abnormality or lump is detected during pregnancy, it should be presented immediately to a physician who will conduct a thorough clinical breast exam. The physician may also order an ultrasound (sonogram) exam or a mammogram or may be both. In many cases, a non-surgical biopsy will be performed if a suspicious breast lump or abnormality is detected in a pregnant woman. A biopsy helps determine whether a breast mass is cancerous or benign. Fine needle aspiration biopsy (FNA) involves using a thin needle to drain fluid or sample cells from the breast. FNA is often used to identify and drain cysts or remove cells for microscopic examination. Other methods of breast biopsy that use larger needles than FNA, such as core needle biopsy or vacuum-assisted biopsy, can also be performed safely during pregnancy if they are warranted. In some cases, an open surgical biopsy may be necessary to diagnose a breast mass. If so, careful planning can help reduce any risks to the mother and fetus.

Breast cancer risk increases with age; therefore, women who delay childbearing gradually move into a higher risk category for the disease. Since many women are delaying childbearing for educational, professional, or personal reasons the number of women who will undergo breast cancer treatment before completing childbearing is increasing

## Effect of subsequent pregnancy on breast carcinoma

Breast carcinoma is not in itself a contraindication to subsequent pregnancy. Pregnancy does not appear to compromise the survival of women with a prior history of breast cancer. No damaging effects on the fetus from maternal breast cancer have been demonstrated, and there are no reported cases of maternal-fetal transfer of breast cancer cells.

The available literature shows that breast cancer patients who subsequently become pregnant have good survival rates. It is generally recommended that patients wait 2 years after diagnosis before attempting to conceive. This allows early recurrence to become manifest, which may influence the decision to become pregnant.

## Chapter 11
# Types of Treatment

The choice of initial treatment depends on the extent to which the spread has occurred. It can be an early breast cancer or locally advanced breast cancer.

The oldest record of breast cancer dates back to 1600 BC. In 1862,[92] Edwin Smith, an American Egyptologist, discovered a 4.68 metre long papyrus describing at least one breast tumor.

- Early Egypt: Treatment was cauterization of the diseased tissue, surgery without anesthesia or antiseptic
- Greece: (130-200 AD) Treatments included special diets, exorcisms and topical applications
- Europe: (14th to 16th century) Andreas Vesalius, a Flemish anatomist, recommended mastectomy and sutures to control the bleeding
- 1685-1770: The physician LeDran was the first to associate the severity of extreme cases of the disease with the spread of cancer to the lymph nodes or under-arm glands
- Mid-1800s: Mastectomies were common, indicating that doctors at the time were aware that the disease could spread
- Late-1800s: Radical mastectomies were often carried out, including the removal of the auxiliary nodes, but usually only for advanced cancers. Patients would generally only survive for three years
- 1930-1950: Physicians began to classify the stage of the cancer

- 1950: Survival rates following mastectomies increases from 10 to 50 per cent
- 1975: Researchers at the University of California discover that certain normal genes somehow become abnormal causing cancer

## Surgery [93]

Most women with breast cancer have some type of surgery. Operations for local treatment include breast-conserving surgery, mastectomy, and axillary (armpit) lymph node sampling and removal. In addition, women may decide to have breast reconstruction at the same time they have the mastectomy, or later on.

## Breast conservation therapy

Lumpectomy removes only the breast lump and a surrounding margin of normal tissue. If examination of the tissue removed by lumpectomy finds there is cancer at the edge of the piece of tissue removed (margin), the surgeon may need to remove additional tissue. This operation is called a re-excision. Radiation therapy is usually given at some time after a lumpectomy. If there is to be chemotherapy, the radiation is usually delayed until the chemotherapy is no longer being given.

## Partial or segmental mastectomy or quadrantectomy

Removes more breast tissue than a lumpectomy (up to one-quarter of the breast). Radiation therapy is usually given after surgery.

Side effects of these operations include temporary swelling and tenderness and hardness due to scar tissue that forms in the surgical site.

For most women with stage I or II of breast cancer, breast conservation therapy (lumpectomy and radiation therapy) is as effective as mastectomy. Survival rates of women treated with these 2 approaches are the same. However, breast conservation therapy is not an option for all women with breast cancer.

Radiation therapy as a part of breast-conserving therapy can sometimes be omitted. Women who may consider lumpectomy without radiation therapy have all of the following:

- Age 70 years or older
- A tumor 2 cm or less that has been completely removed
- A tumor that contains hormone receptors
- No lymph node involvement

## Mastectomy

In a simple or total mastectomy the surgeon removes the entire breast, including the nipple, but does not remove underarm lymph nodes or muscle tissue from beneath the breast. This operation is sometimes used to treat stage 0 breast cancers.

### Modified radical mastectomy

Modified radical mastectomy involves the removal of the entire breast and some of the axillary (underarm) lymph nodes. This is the most common surgery for women with breast cancer who are having the whole breast removed.

### Radical mastectomy

Radical mastectomy is an extensive operation removing the entire breast, axillary lymph nodes, and the pectoral (chest wall) muscles under the breast. This surgery was once very common but because of the disfigurement and side effects it causes and because modified radical mastectomy has been proven to be as effective as radical mastectomy, it is rarely done.

Possible side effects of mastectomy and lumpectomy include wound infection, hematoma (accumulation of blood in the wound), and seroma (accumulation of clear fluid in the wound).

## Choosing between lumpectomy and mastectomy

The advantage of lumpectomy is that it saves the appearance of the breast. A disadvantage is the need for several weeks of radiation therapy after surgery. However, a small percentage of women who have a mastectomy still need radiation therapy to the breast area.

In determining the preference for lumpectomy or mastectomy, be sure to obtain all the facts. Though you may have an initial gut feeling for mastectomy to 'take it all out as quickly as possible,' the fact is that doing so does not provide any better chance of long term survival or a better outcome from treatment in most cases. Large research studies with thousands of women participating and over 20 years of accumulated information show that when lumpectomy can be performed, mastectomy does not provide any better chance of survival from breast cancer than lumpectomy. It is because of these facts that most women do not have the breast removed.

Although most women and their doctors prefer lumpectomy and radiation therapy, your choice will depend on a number of factors, such as:

- How you feel about losing your breast
- How far you have to travel for radiation therapy
- Whether you are willing to have more surgery to reconstruct your breast after having a mastectomy
- Your preference for mastectomy as a way to get rid of all your cancer as quickly as possible

Lumpectomy or breast conservation therapy is usually not recommended for:

- Women who have already had radiation therapy to the affected breast
- Women with two or more areas of cancer in the same breast that are too far apart to be removed through one surgical incision
- Women whose initial lumpectomy along with re-excision has not completely removed the cancer

## Types of Treatment

- Women with certain serious connective tissue diseases such as scleroderma, which make them especially sensitive to the side effects of radiation therapy
- Pregnant women who would require radiation while still pregnant (risking harm to the fetus)
- Women with a tumor larger than 5 cm (2 inches) that doesn't shrink very much with chemotherapy
- Women with cancer that is large relative to a smaller-sized breast

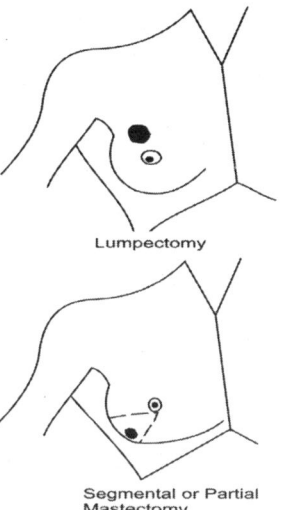

Lumpectomy

Segmental or Partial Mastectomy

## Surgical treatments for breast cancer[93]

### Axillary lymph node dissection

To determine if the breast cancer has spread to axillary (underarm) lymph nodes, some of these lymph nodes are removed (in an operation called axillary dissection) and examined under the microscope.

As noted previously, axillary lymph node dissection is part of a radical or modified radical mastectomy procedure and is usually combined with a breast-conserving procedure such as lumpectomy. Anywhere from about 10 to 40 lymph nodes are removed during axillary lymph node dissection.

Whether or not cancer cells are present in the lymph nodes under the arm is an important factor in selecting adjuvant therapy. It was once believed that removing as many lymph nodes as possible would reduce the risk of spread to other parts of the body and improve the chance of curing the cancer.

It is now known that breast cancer cells that have spread beyond the breast and axillary lymph nodes are best treated by systemic therapy. Axillary dissection is used as a test to help guide other breast cancer treatment decisions.

The main side effect of removing axillary lymph nodes is lymph edema (swelling of the arm). About 10% to 30% of women who have underarm lymph nodes removed develop lymphedema. If your arm is swollen, tight, or painful after lymph node surgery, be sure to tell someone in your cancer care team promptly.

You may also have temporary or permanent limitations in arm and shoulder movement after surgery. Numbness of the upper inner arm skin is another common side effect because the nerve controlling this skin sensation travels through the lymph node area.

## Sentinel lymph node biopsy (SLNB)

Although lymph node dissection is a safe operation and has low rates of serious side effects, doctors have developed another way of learning if cancer has spread to lymph nodes without removing all of them first. This procedure is called the 'sentinel lymph node biopsy'.

In this procedure the surgeon finds and removes the 'sentinel node'—the first lymph node into which a tumor drains, and the one most likely to contain cancer cells. The surgeon injects a radioactive substance and/or a blue dye into the area around the tumor. Lymphatic vessels carry these substances into the sentinel node and provide the doctor with a 'lymph node map'. The doctor can either see the blue dye or detect the radioactivity with a Geiger counter. He/she then removes the node or nodes (often 2 or 3) for examination by the pathologist.

If the sentinel node(s) contains cancer, the surgeon will perform an axillary dissection—removal of more lymph nodes in the armpit. This may be done at the same time or several days after the original sentinel node biopsy. The timing of the axillary dissection depends on how easily the cancer can be seen in the lymph node at the time of surgery. Sometimes it is obvious and at other times it will only be found by thorough microscopic study by a pathologist.

If the sentinel node is cancer-free, the patient will not need more lymph node surgery and can avoid the side effects of full lymph node surgery.

This limited sampling of lymph nodes is not always appropriate. It is most suitable if there is a single tumor less than 5 cm in the breast, no prior chemotherapy or hormone therapy has been given, and the lymph nodes do not feel enlarged.

Sentinel lymph node biopsy is a complex technique that requires a great deal of skill. Therefore, doctors recommend that sentinel lymph node biopsy be done only by a team known to have experience with this technique. If you are considering having such a biopsy, ask your health care team if this is something they do regularly.

## Reconstructive surgery and breast implant surgery

These procedures are not done to treat cancer but to restore the breast's appearance after mastectomy. If you are going to have a mastectomy and are thinking about having reconstruction immediately, it's important to consult with a plastic surgeon who is an expert in breast reconstruction before the surgery.

Decisions about the type of reconstruction and when it will be done depends on each woman's medical situation and personal preferences. Your breast can be reconstructed at the same time as the mastectomy (immediate reconstruction) or at a later time (delayed reconstruction). Reconstruction may use implants and/or tissue from other parts of your body (autologous tissue reconstruction).

For many, the thought of surgery can be very frightening. But with a better understanding of what to expect before, during and after the operation, many fears can be relieved.

## Before surgery

You usually meet with your surgeon a few days before the operation to discuss the procedure. This is a good time to ask specific questions about the surgery and review potential risks. You will be asked to sign a consent form, giving the doctor permission to perform the surgery. Take your time and review the form carefully to be certain that you understand what you are signing.

Sometimes, doctors send material for you to review in prior to of your appointment, so you will have plenty of time to read it and won't feel rushed. You may also be asked to give consent for researchers to use any tissue or blood that is not needed for diagnostic purposes. Although this may not be of direct use to you, it may be very helpful to women in the future.

You may be asked to donate blood before some operations, such as a mastectomy combined with natural tissue reconstruction, if the doctors think a transfusion might be needed. You might feel more secure knowing that if a transfusion is needed, you will receive your own blood. If you do not receive your own blood, it is important you know that in the United States, blood transfusion from another person is nearly as safe as receiving your own blood. Ask your doctor about your possible need for a blood transfusion.

Your doctor will review your medical records and ask you about any medicines you are taking. This is to be sure that you are not taking anything that will interfere with the surgery. For example, if you are taking a blood-thinning medicine (even aspirin), you may be asked to stop taking the drug about a week or two before the surgery. Usually, you will be told not to eat or drink anything for 8 to 12 hours before the surgery, especially if you are going to have general anesthesia (will be 'asleep' during surgery).

You will also meet with the anesthesiologist who will be giving you the anesthesia during your surgery. The type of anesthesia used depends largely on the kind of surgery being done and your medical history.

General anesthesia is usually given whenever the surgery involves a mastectomy or an axillary node dissection. You will be given an IV (intravenous) line to give medications that may be needed during the surgery. Usually you will be hooked up to an electrocardiogram

(ECG) machine and have a blood pressure cuff on your arm, so your heart rhythm and blood pressure can be checked during the surgery.

## Surgery

For your surgery, you may be offered the choice of an outpatient procedure or you may be admitted to the hospital. How long you stay in the hospital depends on the surgery being performed, your overall state of health and whether you have any other medical problems, how well you do during the surgery, and how you feel after the surgery. Decisions about the length of your stay should be made by you and your doctor and not dictated by what your insurance will pay, but it is important to check your insurance coverage before surgery.

As a general rule, women having a mastectomy and/or axillary lymph node dissection stay in the hospital for 1 or 2 nights and then go home. However, some women may be placed in a 23-hour, short-stay observation unit before going home. In this situation, care is continued at home with a home care nurse visiting you to monitor and provide care.

Lumpectomy and sentinel lymph node biopsy are usually done in an outpatient surgery center, and an overnight stay in the hospital is usually not necessary.

The length of the operation depends on the type of surgery being done. For example, a mastectomy with axillary lymph node dissection will take from 2 to 3 hours. After your surgery, you will be taken to the recovery room, where you will stay until you are awake and your condition and vital signs (blood pressure, pulse, and breathing) are stable.

## After surgery

You will have a dressing (bandage) over the surgery site. You may have one or more drains (plastic or rubber tubes) from the breast or underarm area to remove blood and lymph fluid that collects during the healing process. Care of the drains includes emptying and measuring the fluid and identifying problems the doctor or nurse needs to know

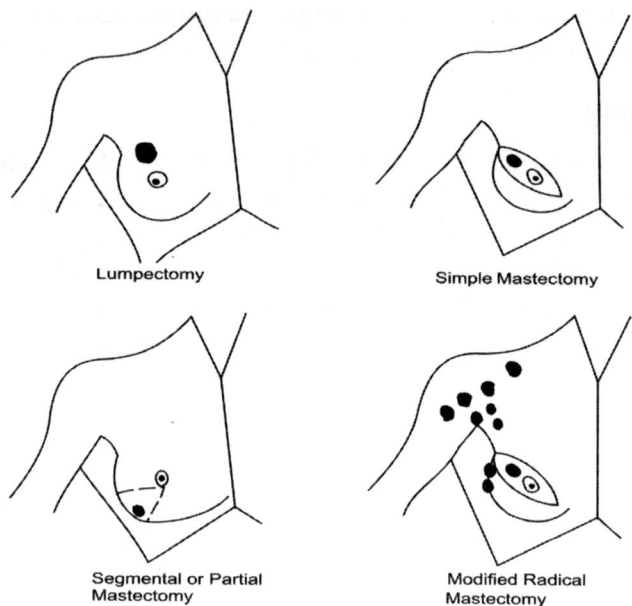

Lumpectomy

Simple Mastectomy

Segmental or Partial Mastectomy

Modified Radical Mastectomy

about. Most drains stay in place for 1 or 2 weeks. When drainage has decreased to about 30 cc (1 fluid ounce) each day, often the drain will be removed.

Doctors rarely put the arm in a sling to hold it in place. Most doctors will want you to start moving the arm so that it won't get stiff. Women who have a lumpectomy or mastectomy are surprised by how little pain they have in the breast area. But they are less happy with the strange sensations (numbness, pinching/pulling feeling) in the underarm area.

Care of the surgery site and arm should be discussed with your doctor. Written instructions about care after surgery are usually given to you and your caregivers. These instructions should include:

- The care of the surgical wound and dressing
- How to monitor drainage and take care of the drains
- How to recognize signs of infection
- When to call the doctor or nurse

- When to begin using the arm and how to do arm exercises to prevent stiffness
- When to resume wearing a bra
- When to begin using a prosthesis and what type to use (after mastectomy)
- What to eat and not to eat
- Use of medications, including pain medicines
- Any restrictions of activity
- What to expect regarding sensations or numbness in the breast and arm
- What to expect regarding feelings about body image

Most patients see their doctor within 7 to 14 days following the surgery. Your doctor should explain the results of your pathology report and talk to you about the need for further treatment. If you will need more treatment, you will be referred to a medical oncologist and/or radiation oncologist.[93]

## Chemotherapy

Chemotherapy actually just means treatment with drugs. But we use it commonly to mean 'cytotoxic chemotherapy'—treatment with drugs that kill cells. Chemotherapy uses these cytotoxic drugs to destroy cancer cells. The drugs work by disrupting the growth of cancer cells. As they circulate in the blood, they can reach them wherever they are in your body.

The drugs can't tell the difference between cancer cells and normal cells. They just kill cells that are actively growing and dividing into new cells. Cancer cells do this much more often than normal cells, so they are more at risk from the treatment. For breast cancer, you may have chemotherapy:
- Before surgery: to shrink a tumor down (neoadjuvant therapy)
- After surgery: to reduce the chance of it spreading or coming back (adjuvant therapy)

- As treatment for breast cancer that has spread or come back

## Treatment before surgery

Chemotherapy before surgery can make a tumor smaller. This can mean you need less surgery. For example, you may be able to just have the cancer removed instead of having a mastectomy. In rare cases, women do not need breast surgery at all after neoadjuvant chemotherapy, as there is no longer any sign of cancer. But they may still need to have some lymph nodes removed from the armpit.

Your specialist may suggest neoadjuvant chemotherapy because he or she thinks it may help to stop your breast cancer coming back.

## Treatment after surgery

Chemotherapy after surgery is called adjuvant therapy. You may have this treatment because:

- The lymph nodes under your arm contained breast cancer cells
- You had a large primary cancer in the breast
- Your breast cancer cells were of high grade (grade 3)
- Your cancer cells did not test positive for hormone receptors and so are not likely to respond well to hormone therapy

Doctors use adjuvant therapy when they think there is a significant risk that cancer cells have broken away from the tumor in the breast and spread before you had it removed. So, there may be cancer cells elsewhere in your body. Adjuvant therapy can kill these cells off and so reduces the risk of the cancer coming back.

If you are still having periods, chemotherapy may help in another way. It can stop your ovaries from making estrogen. Estrogen can stimulate your breast cancer to grow. Some specialists think this may be the main reason why chemotherapy is such a successful adjuvant treatment in pre-menopausal women. Unfortunately, the loss of estrogen will mean you may have an early menopause and are infertile. This is not always the case. Some women do find that their ovaries begin working again after chemotherapy. This depends on your age when you are treated and on the chemotherapy drugs that you are given. If you are still not having periods a year after your treatment finished, then unfortunately, it is not likely that your ovaries will recover.

## Treating cancer that has come back

Many women have no more problems after their original treatment for breast cancer. But sometimes breast cancer does come back or spread. This is called 'secondary breast cancer' or 'metastatic breast cancer'. If the breast cancer comes back in the same breast it is called 'local recurrence'. Secondary breast cancer is often treated with chemotherapy.

Remember, secondary breast cancer can often be kept under control with the right treatment.

You may take some chemotherapy drugs by mouth but you have to have most of them injected into a vein.

You have chemotherapy as a course of treatment. The length of time the course takes will vary considerably depending on the drugs you are having. Usually, you have the drugs for one to five days, then have a break for three to four weeks. The drug treatment, followed by the break makes up one 'cycle'. Then the cycle begins again. You have up to eight treatment cycles. So a complete course of treatment can take up to eight months.

The number of courses you will have depends on:

- The type of cancer
- The drugs used
- In 'metastatic' breast cancer it will also depend on how well the cancer responds to the drugs.

You are most likely to have your chemotherapy treatment in the out patients' department. But you may have to spend a few days in the hospital. This depends on the drugs you have. Each time you start a new cycle of treatment, your doctors will want to check your blood cell counts first. They need to do this to make sure you have recovered from your last chemotherapy. In practice, this usually just means getting there earlier and spending a while hanging about for the results. But if your blood counts are not high enough, your chemotherapy may be delayed for a few days.

Very high doses of chemotherapy have been tried for breast cancer. This means such high doses that it damages your bone marrow. So you have to have some bone marrow or blood stem cells collected first and then given back to you after the chemotherapy. This type of chemotherapy is still experimental. In trials so far, this treatment hasn't been any better than regular chemotherapy for breast cancer. And it is considerably more risky.

## Breast reconstruction

Despite an increasing trend towards conservative surgery, women still require mastectomy. These women can now be offered immediate or delayed reconstruction of the breast. Most common type of reconstruction is using saline implants under pectoralis major muscle (chest). However patients require counseling before this procedure so that their expectation of cosmetic outcome is not unrealistic.

Surgery, radiotherapy, chemotherapy and hormonal therapy are the major treatment modalities available.

## Drugs

There are quite a few chemotherapy drugs commonly used for breast cancer. So we can't say what your doctor will recommend. Usually you would have a combination of about 3 chemotherapy drugs together. But in some circumstances, your specialist may suggest one on its own. The drugs are:

- Cyclophosphamide
- Epirubicin
- 5-Fluorouracil or 5 FU

- Methotrexate
- Mitomycin
- Mitozantrone (mitoxantrone)
- Doxorubicin (Adriamycin)
- Docetaxel (Taxotere)

Some of the commonest combinations used for breast cancer are:

- CMF - Cyclophosphamide, methotrexate and 5-FU
- FEC - Epirubicin, cyclophosphamide and 5-FU
- E-CMF - Epirubicin, followed by CMF
- AC - Doxorubicin (adriamycin) and cyclophosphamide
- MMM - Methotrexate, mitozantrone and mitomycin
- MM - Methotrexate and mitozantrone

The adjuvant chemotherapy for breast cancer should consist of 4 to 8 cycles of a combination of drugs, including an anthracycline (epirubicin or doxorubicin).

Different combinations of drugs have different side effects.[94]

## Taking supplements with chemotherapy

There is increasing concern amongst doctors about dietary supplements and herbal medicines. Doctors often don't know what their patients are buying over the counter or getting from alternative or complementary therapy practitioners. There is nothing wrong with trying to help yourself get better, of course. But we don't know enough scientifically about how some supplements may interact with chemotherapy.

Talk to your specialist about any other tablets or medicines you take while you are on active treatment. It may not be a good idea to take anything that claims to boost your immune system, for instance.

Good self-care during chemotherapy (treatment with anti-cancer drugs) will help offset some of the side effects you may experience. Save your energy for healing by planning ahead for the basics, such as grocery shopping and getting to your appointments.

## Steps

Research as much as you can about your condition. The more you know, the less you will fear the unknown.

Have any needed dental work done before you begin treatment. Buy a new toothbrush, and plan to buy one after each monthly cycle of chemotherapy to prevent buildup of bacterial or chemical residue.

Consider cutting your hair shorter if your physician has confirmed that you will lose your hair. This will ease you into having less hair.

Shop for a wig before your treatment begins, if you plan to wear one, taking your time to find a colour and length that goes well with your personality and physical characteristics.

Organize your nutritional needs ahead of time and have your refrigerator and pantry stocked with low-fat, low-sugar snacks, plus lots of green leafy vegetables and fresh fruit. If you don't already, plan to eat three meals a day during treatment.

Buy or borrow books and tapes ahead of time to take with you for the waiting room and treatment.

Remember to stock up on water and other fluids to take with you to each treatment so you avoid dehydration. Also, carry mints or sugar-free hard candy with you.

Wear loose, comfortable clothing to each appointment.

## Tips and warnings

i. Take notes at doctor's appointments, and keep a running list of questions for your health care provider.
ii. Keep a daily journal during treatment to better understand your feelings and the treatment process. This will also bring to the

surface any questions you may need to ask your physician.

iii. Learn some muscle relaxation exercises ahead of time so you can practice them during your treatment. Try relaxing and tensing the muscles of one of your legs, starting with your toes and working your way up your leg. Hold your breath each time you become tense, breathing out as you relax. Next, work your way up your other leg. Finally, relax other muscle groups, working all the way up your body to the top of your head.

iv. Stay away from fatty foods, as weight gain is more common than most people expect with the new anti-nausea drugs available to patients undergoing chemotherapy.

## Radiation therapy

Radiation therapy is offered to breast cancer patients to rid the body of any microscopic cancer cells that may remain near the area where the cancer was originally found. The usual course of therapy includes daily treatments five days a week for five to seven weeks. Each session generally lasts an hour or less.

Radiation therapy works by causing changes at the molecular level in tissues where the radiation beam is targeted. Giving all the radiation needed at one time would cause significant and irreparable damage not only to cancer cells, but also to normal cells. However, giving small doses of radiation each day enables the majority of healthy cells to repair any damage, while rendering cancer cells inactive. The radiation oncologist is the medical doctor in charge of a patient's radiation treatment. He or she prescribes and plans the radiation course that patients will be taking. He/she will also be monitoring patients while they are undergoing treatment and will be providing individualized quality care. Any side effects from the radiation will be recognized and treated by the radiation oncologist. The other members of the medical team include the medical physicist, the radiation therapist and the dosimeterist.

The job of the medical physicist is to ensure the proper running of the machinery and perform regular calibrations and checks of the machine that will deliver the radiation.

The radiation therapist is the person who delivers the radiation each day and will be working under the orders and the prescription of the radiation oncologist.

The dosimeterist calculates the doses of radiation at various points in the body.

Patients may also encounter a registered nurse, dietician, and social worker, during their course of treatment. These individuals will play a big role in the overall care.

The goal of radiation can be:

- Curative or radical
- Palliative, that is, to reduce symptoms of pain
- Adjuvant which is a treatment that is dietician to reduce the risk of tumor recurrence. Radiation can be used after surgery for breast cancer in order to reduce the risk of the cancer returning

There are basically two types of radiation treatment:

- External radiation
- Brachytherapy, or radiation at a short distance
- A patient may receive one or the other, or a combination of both

## Steps in radiation treatment

**Consultation:** At the beginning, the patient will be seen by the radiation oncologist for a consultation. During the consultation, the radiation oncologist will perform a history and a physical examination. He will review all the pertinent data and all of the investigations that have been performed. He may also request other tests or consultations to be made.

**Simulation:** The next step is simulation or treatment planning. After the consultation, the radiation oncologist will formulate a treatment

## Types of Treatment

plan. Here, the patient comes to the radiation department and lies down on a table under a machine, called a simulator. Various immobilization devices may be necessary, such as a head rest or a face mask, in order to make sure the patient is positioned correctly and in the same way for each treatment. There will be various markings that will be made on the skin and various x-rays will be taken.

Photographs may also be taken and this will help the radiation therapist to deliver the treatment on subsequent days. Remember that patients may require more than one session for simulation. Simulation is very important, since it is the step that allows for proper planning and delivery of the actual treatment. After simulation, there is a lot of behind-the-scenes work. Here the medical physicist and dosimeterist are involved. CT scans may have to be taken in order that the computers can calculate and prescribe the dose distribution of the radiation.

Blocks and shields are often fashioned for the patient undergoing radiation treatment. Blocks or shields are pieces of lead that are placed on a tray between the patient and the treatment machine. The blocks basically will cover up normal tissues in the body in order that radiation is delivered principally to the tumor. External radiation is a safe and basically painless form of treatment.

### Treatment

Usually, the treatment course lasts between two and five weeks. Patients are brought by the radiation therapist into the treatment room and positioned onto the treatment table. The treatment will then be set up by the radiation therapist, and the actual treatment itself will only last a couple of minutes. During the actual treatment, patients are alone in the room but the radiation therapist is outside and can hear patients through a close circuit television.

The treatment is painless. Patients do not hear or feel anything during or after the treatment. Patients will then return on schedule to complete the treatment course. During the radiation course, patients are monitored by the radiation oncologist and his/her staff. These are called status checks.

Patients should inform the radiation oncologist of any new symptoms. The side effects of the radiation depend on the exact type of tumor treated and the location of the radiation treatment. During the course of treatment, patients will undergo blood tests, sometimes once a week and they will also have port films performed. These are x-ray pictures taken on the treatment machine which are used to ascertain the accuracy of the treatment plan.

Radiation works best when it is given in small doses over several sessions. In this way, it can kill the tumor cells and yet allow sufficient time for the normal healthy cells around the tumor to repair any damage from the radiation

## External beam radiation

This is the usual type of radiation therapy for women with breast cancer. The radiation is focused from a machine outside the body on the area affected by the cancer. This usually includes the whole breast and depending on the size and extent of the cancer, may include the chest wall and underarm area as well. Radiation therapy is much like getting a diagnostic x-ray but the radiation is more intense. The procedure itself is painless.

Before your treatments start, the radiation team carefully takes measurements to determine the correct angles for aiming the radiation beams and the proper dose of radiation. They will make some ink marks or small tattoos on your skin that they will use it later as a guide to focus the radiation on the right area. Patients who receive breast radiation after lumpectomy are usually treated five days a week in an outpatient center for about six or seven weeks, with each treatment lasting a few minutes.

A new technique to give radiation over a much shorter period of time (five days total) and to only the part of the breast with the cancer is currently being done in clinical research trials. This is called partial breast irradiation. It is hoped that partial breast irradiation will prove to be equal to the current, standard whole breast irradiation. However, partial breast irradiation is still experimental.

Lotions, powders, deodorants, and antiperspirants can interfere with external beam radiation therapy, so you should avoid using them until treatments are complete.

The main side effects of external beam radiation therapy are swelling and heaviness in the breast, sunburn-like skin changes in the treated area, and fatigue. You should avoid exposing the treated skin to the sun because it can make the skin changes worse. These changes to the breast tissue and skin usually go away in 6 to 12 months. There may also be some aching in the breast and rarely, a rib fracture related to radiation therapy.

In some women, the breast becomes smaller and firmer after radiation therapy. Radiation therapy of axillary lymph nodes also can cause lymphedema. Radiation therapy is not given during pregnancy because it can harm the fetus.

## Brachytherapy

Brachytherapy is radiation at short distances. The source of radiation is made in the form of wires, seeds or plaques and are inserted into the tumor for delivering high doses of radiation. These radioactive sources are Cesium, Iridium and Iodine. This type of treatment is very effective in certain types of cancer, such as cancer of the cervix, certain forms of head and neck cancer and lung cancer.

## Intra-cavity radiation

Here the radioactive sources are placed in a holder and inserted into the body organ, such as the uterus, or into the vagina.

## Interstitial therapy

Here rods, ribbons, or wires are directly inserted into the soft tissues of the body and placed right into the tumor.

With these two types of treatment, patients would most likely be admitted to the hospital and have the procedure done during an operation and under anesthesia. Patients would most likely remain in the hospital for several days while the radiation source is in place. In a few instances, the source will be left permanently inside the body. However, in the majority of cases, the radioactive sources will be removed after a few days. Patients will have restrictions in the number of people visiting and the time of visitation.

## High dose rate brachytherapy

This is another form of radiation therapy that has become very popular in recent years. This is an outpatient form of radiation treatment. The high dose rate machine contains a very high activity radiation source and the source is then delivered through a catheter into a particular organ that is harboring the cancer. Usually the treatment itself lasts only a few minutes. Thereafter, the source is removed and stored within the machine and the patients go home. Patients may require several sessions of high-dose rate brachytherapy in order to derive the maximum benefit. Many patients will experience side effects from radiation.

Radiation therapy is a treatment with high-energy rays or particles that destroy cancer cells. This treatment may be used to destroy cancer cells that remain in the breast, chest wall or underarm area after surgery. Radiation may also be needed after mastectomy in cases with either a cancer larger than 5 cm in size or when cancer is found in the lymph nodes.

In some cases, the area treated by radiation therapy may also include supraclavicular lymph nodes (nodes above the collarbone) and internal mammary lymph nodes (nodes beneath the sternum or breast bone in the center of the chest). When given after surgery, radiation therapy is usually not started until the tissues have been able to heal for about a month. Radiation therapy is usually delayed until chemotherapy is complete.

The extent of radiation depends on whether or not a lumpectomy or mastectomy was performed and whether or not lymph nodes are involved. If a lumpectomy was done, the entire breast receives radiation and an extra boost of radiation is given to the area in the breast where the cancer was removed to prevent it from coming back in that area.

## Points to remember about radiation therapy

i. The actual delivery of radiation treatment is painless. But the radiation itself does cause some pain and discomfort over time.
ii. External radiation treatment, the most common kind of radiation therapy, does not make you radioactive.
iii. You will receive treatment five days a week for up to seven weeks. Occasionally, radiation may be given twice a day over one week.
iv. Since the daily appointments are usually for about half an hour, you will most likely be able to keep to your normal routine during your course of treatment.
v. You will not lose your hair when you are undergoing radiation therapy, unless you are also being treated with chemotherapy.
vi. Your skin in the area where you are receiving radiation can turn red, become more sensitive, and get easily irritated.
vii. Over the course of your treatment, you may begin to feel tired. This feeling can last for a few weeks, even months–after treatment ends.
viii. The side effects of radiation treatment are usually temporary.
ix. For most types of breast cancer, radiation therapy after surgery significantly decreases the possibility of cancer recurrence.

Radiation therapy is usually used with:
- Chemotherapy (medicine used to destroy cancer cells)
- Surgery to remove the cancer

You should ask your health care provider about these treatments. You may choose not to have treatment but you should ask your health care provider how this may increase your risk. Also ask your radiation oncologist how the radiation will affect you

## How should I prepare for this procedure?

Follow the instructions provided by the radiation therapist and the radiation therapy technologists. Do not use creams, powders, or deodorants unless they say it is okay. You should wear clothes that are easy to take off and that do not rub the treated area.

## What happens during the procedure?

First you will need to take off the clothing covering your chest. The radiation therapy technologist will ask you to lie on a treatment table and raise your arms over your head. The therapist will use the ink marks he/she made on you at an earlier visit to make sure the radiation is aimed at the correct place(s).

If you have had your breast removed, you may have a bolus (a cold, rubber like mat) placed on top of your chest. The therapist will help you lie in the correct position and leave you alone in the treatment room. She or he will watch you on a TV monitor and you can talk with the therapist over an intercom. You will hear the radiation machine buzz for about 30 seconds as it sends radiation to the specific area marked on your body. You may have one or more of these treatments done from other angles.

The treatment is painless. Each session takes between 15 and 30 minutes. When the session is over, the therapist will help you off the table and you may go home.

You will receive radiation therapy five days a week for four to seven weeks. During the weeks of treatment the therapist weighs you and may do tests, such as blood cell counts, to check the effect the radiation is having on your body.

## What happens after the procedure?

You should talk with your radiation oncologist and the staff about your diet, caring for your skin, and ways to care for yourself. The skin in the treatment area may become red. It may feel like sunburn. Also, you may lose hair in the treatment area. Check first with the radiation therapist before you use any drugs or products such as shampoo or makeup while you are getting radiation treatment. You may notice you do not feel like eating. You may also find you need more rest as you have more treatments.

Try to keep your arms limber. They may be sore. The therapist will give you some exercises to help your arms move easily. You should protect your skin from the sun by keeping it covered with clothing.

After your last session, the staff will wipe off the ink marks on your body. Even though you will no longer be receiving treatments, the radiation keeps acting on the cancer for several weeks. The side effects of the radiation should go away a few weeks after the end of the therapy.

Your breast may feel firm or change in size. You should continue to perform breast self-exams. You should take special care of the arm on the side of the treatment, trying to avoid hurting or stressing it.

Ask your radiation oncologist how active you can be and how often you should return to the radiation and oncology clinic for checkups. Keep on seeing your regular health care provider for your other health care needs.

## What are the benefits of this procedure?

The cancer may be destroyed or slowed down.

## What are the risks associated with this procedure?

- There is a risk of hurting the healthy cells or forming scar tissue
- Your skin could be hurt or get darker

- Your arm on the side of treatment may swell. It may become infected more easily.
- If you are having both radiation therapy and chemotherapy, you may have more side effects.
- The radiation therapy may not destroy all the cancer.
- The cancer may come back

You should ask your health care provider how these risks apply to you.

### When should I call the health care provider?

Call your health care provider immediately if:

- You get fever
- You have unexpected pain
- You develop swelling in your arm

## Hormone therapy

Hormones are substances that occur naturally in the body where they control the growth and activity of normal cells. Although they do not usually affect cancer cells, in breast cancer the situation is different.

The female hormones, estrogen and progesterone are naturally produced by the ovaries before menopause. After the menopause, estrogen is made in much smaller amounts by small glands above the kidneys, called the adrenal glands. These hormones affect the growth of some breast cancer cells. This means that drugs or treatments that block the effects of hormones, or lower the levels of estrogen and progesterone, can be used as a treatment for some types of breast cancer. Hormone therapy is another form of adjuvant systemic therapy. The hormone estrogen is produced mainly by a woman's ovaries until menopause. After menopause it is made mostly in the body's fat tissue, where a testosterone-like hormone made by the adrenal gland is converted into estrogen. Estrogen promotes the growth of about two thirds of breast cancers (those containing estrogen or progesterone receptors and called hormone receptor positive cancers). Due to this, several approaches to blocking the effect of estrogen or lowering estrogen levels are used to treat breast cancer.

You may have hormone therapy to treat breast cancer:

- Before breast surgery
- After breast surgery
- That has spread or come back after it was first treated.

## Does everyone have hormone therapy?

Hormone therapy isn't always a suitable treatment for breast cancer. You will have tests on your cancer cells to see if they have hormone receptors. These are areas that allow estrogen or progesterone to lock onto the cell. The hormone then stimulates the cancer cell to grow. Your cancer cells can be tested for estrogen receptors (ER) or progesterone receptors (PR). If you have neither, your specialist may suggest you have chemotherapy after surgery instead of hormone therapy.

## Before surgery

You may have hormone therapy to shrink a cancer in the breast before surgery. This can mean that you need a smaller operation than you otherwise would. It may mean you can have just the cancer removed, rather than needing a mastectomy. Hormone therapy may also help to stop the cancer coming back after your operation.

## After surgery

This is the commonest time to have hormone therapy for breast cancer. Hormone treatment has been proved to reduce the risk of breast cancer coming back. Hormone therapy seems to work best for women who have estrogen receptor positive cancers. You have the treatment for some years after your diagnosis. Exactly for how long, depends on the treatment you are having. Tamoxifen is usually prescribed for five years.

One advantage of hormone treatments is that hormones are very safe to take and although side effects can occasionally be troublesome, they are rarely serious.

## Types of hormone therapy

There are several types of hormone drugs used for primary breast cancer including

- Tamoxifen
- Aromatase inhibitors
- Pituitary downregulators

## Tamoxifen

This is a common and very successful hormone treatment for breast cancer. It is the drug you are most likely to take for five years after breast cancer surgery. Tamoxifen has made a major contribution to the treatment of breast cancer. It is a relatively safe drug and most women have few problems with it although it does have some side effects. Doctors may now sometimes prescribe aromatase inhibitors as an alternative to tamoxifen, or following tamoxifen for some women with breast cancer.

## Aromatase inhibitors

Although women who past their menopause do not produce estrogen from their ovaries, a small amount is produced by the adrenal glands (small glands above the kidneys). Aromatase inhibitors block this estrogen from being made. So these drugs are only suitable for women who've had their menopause. Aromatase inhibitors have always been used to treat breast cancer that has spread. Now, some are also licensed to treat women with early breast cancer who have had their menopause.

Anastrozole, exemestane and letrozole are all tablets you take once a day. They can cause hot flushes and may make you feel sick.

## Pituitary downregulators

These are also called LHRH analogues 'luteinising hormone releasing hormone'. It blocks a hormone in the brain that stimulates ovaries to make and release estrogen.

The commonest of these drugs is grosgrain. Because they stop the ovaries from working, doctors use these drugs to treat women who are still having periods. Stopping the ovaries from working is called 'ovarian ablation'. These drugs do stop your ovaries from working, so that you won't have periods or release eggs while you are having the injections. But this is reversible. When you stop taking the drug, your ovaries should start working again. But, if you are close to the age at which your menopause would naturally start, your ovaries may not start working again after this type of treatment. So it can tip you into an early menopause.

You have grosgrain as an injection once a month. There is a three monthly injection but it isn't reliable enough at switching off the ovaries for the whole three months. You are likely to have menopausal symptoms, such as hot flushes and mood changes while you are on grosgrain. There is information on ways of coping with menopausal symptoms in the section on living with breast cancer.

## Other ways of switching off the ovaries

If you do not like the idea of a monthly injection, there are other methods of ovarian ablation. Most young women with breast cancer have chemotherapy that may stop your ovaries from working, but not in all women. If you continue to have periods after your chemotherapy, your doctor may be keen that you have another treatment to stop your ovaries working. Apart from grosgrain, there are two other ways of doing this, but both of them will affect your ovaries permanently. You could have:

- Your ovaries removed in an operation
- A low dose of radiotherapy to your ovaries

Both the surgery and the radiotherapy will cause a sudden menopause.

### Megestrol acetate

Megestrol acetate is a progesterone-like drug used for hormone treatment of advanced breast cancer, usually for women whose cancers do not respond to the other hormone treatments. Its major side effect is weight gain, and it is sometimes used to reverse weight loss in patients with advanced cancer.

### Other ways to control hormones

Androgens (male hormones) may be considered after other hormone treatments for advanced breast cancer have been tried. Androgens cause masculine characteristics to occur, for example, more body hair and a deeper voice. They are sometimes effective.[93]

### Hormone therapy: Cancer treatment for certain hormone-sensitive cancers

People with certain hormone-sensitive cancers may benefit from hormone therapy as part of their cancer treatment. Find out how it works.

The term 'hormone therapy' might make you think of women taking estrogen to reduce their symptoms of menopause or men taking testosterone to slow the effects of ageing. But hormone therapy for cancer which also called endocrine therapy, is something completely different. Hormone therapy for cancer alters the hormones in your body to help control or cure cancer.

Hormone therapies associated with menopause and ageing seek to increase the amount of certain hormones in your body to compensate for age- or disease-related hormonal declines. But hormone therapy as a cancer treatment either reduces the level of specific hormones in your body or alters your cancer's ability to use these hormones to grow and spread.

If your cancer is one that is sensitive to hormones, you might benefit from hormone therapy as part of your cancer treatment. Learn the basics of hormone therapy, how it works as a cancer treatment and its side effects. That way you'll be prepared to discuss it if your doctor recommends it as a cancer treatment option.

## How hormone therapy cancer treatment works

Specific types of tumors like tumors of the breast and of the prostate rely on hormones such as estrogen and testosterone to survive and grow. Hormone therapy is a cancer treatment that attacks these hormone-dependent tumors in two ways:

i. **Reducing hormones in your body:** By reducing the level of estrogen or testosterone in your body, hormone therapy cuts off the supply of hormones your cancer relies on for its survival.

ii. **Changing your cancer's ability to use hormones:** Synthetic hormones can bind to your cancer's hormone receptors, blocking your cancer's ability to get the hormones it needs for growth.

By altering your cancer's hormone supply, hormone therapy can make your tumors shrink. But this cancer treatment only works for hormone-sensitive cancers.

## Who can benefit from hormone therapy cancer treatment?

If your cancer is hormone sensitive, you might benefit from hormone therapy as part of your cancer treatment. Your doctor can tell you whether or not your cancer is sensitive to hormones. This is usually determined by taking a sample of your tumor (biopsy) for analysis in a laboratory.

## Uses of hormone therapy cancer treatment

Hormone therapy is rarely used as a main (primary) cancer treatment. It is usually used in combination with other types of cancer treatments, including surgery, radiation and chemotherapy.

Your doctor might use a hormone therapy before you begin a primary cancer treatment, such as before surgery to remove a tumor. This is called **neoadjuvant therapy**. Hormone therapy can sometimes shrink a tumor to a more manageable size so that it's easier to remove during surgery.

Hormone therapy is sometimes given in addition to the primary treatment, usually after, in an effort to prevent the cancer from recurring (adjuvant therapy). If you've had surgery to remove your tumor and it appears that all of your cancer has been removed, your doctor might use hormone therapy to try to keep your cancer from coming back.

In some cases of advanced (metastatic) cancers, such as in advanced prostate cancer and advanced breast cancer, hormone therapy is sometimes used as the main treatment.

Researchers are also exploring the use of hormone therapies to prevent cancer from occurring in people with a high risk of cancer.

Radiation is used to suppress the production of hormones. Just as is true of surgery, it's used most commonly to stop hormone production in the testicles, ovaries and adrenal and pituitary glands. Your doctor might recommend radiation therapy rather than surgery if surgery is too risky for you or if it carries too many side effects.

Common side effects in men undergoing hormone therapy include:

- Decrease in sexual desire
- Enlarged breasts
- Hot flushes
- Inability to achieve an erection
- Incontinence
- Osteoporosis

In women undergoing hormone therapy, side effects can include symptoms similar to those of menopause, such as:

- Fatigue

- Hot flushes
- Mood swings
- Nausea
- Osteoporosis
- Weight gain

## Resistance to hormone therapy

If you opt for hormone therapy as a cancer treatment, be aware that the effects of hormone therapy may be limited. Most advanced hormone-sensitive cancers eventually become resistant to hormone treatment and find ways to thrive without hormones.

For instance, many women who've had surgery for breast cancer take tamoxifen only for five years because taking it for a longer period doesn't offer any further benefit and may actually increase the risk that cancer will recur. But you're not out of options at the end of those five years. Your doctor may prescribe another form of hormone therapy to which your cancer may respond. Women who've taken tamoxifen may be able to take an aromatase inhibitor, such as letrozole.

If you have prostate cancer, your doctor might prescribe intermittent dosing of hormone therapy drugs in an attempt to prevent your cancer from becoming resistant to therapy. This means you won't take a drug continuously for several years. Instead you'll start and stop taking the drug as your doctor closely monitors your cancer.

## Deciding what's best for you

Talk with your doctor about the potential side effects and the possible benefits of all the treatments you're considering. Balancing the risks with the benefits is the best way to choose a treatment that's best for you.

## Overview

Depending on the type of breast cancer and the stage of disease, a wide range of treatment options are available. These can be undertaken individually or in combination and include the following: Radiation Therapy, Chemotherapy, Hormonal Therapy, High-dose Chemotherapy and Complementary Therapy. Clinical trials may also be an option to be considered.

## Immunotherapy for specific cancers

The FDA has approved several immunotherapies for use against specific cancers.

Many other immunotherapies have shown promising results and are moving through the testing process of phase I, phase II and phase III clinical trials blocking the access of the growth factors to the cancer cells and slowing their growth. Clinical trials of other HER2/neu antibodies are currently underway.

Some interferons and interleukins have shown promise against breast cancer, particularly when used in combination with tumor vaccines or immunotoxins.

Autologous vaccine therapy has lengthened remission and survival times of some women with early breast cancer; this approach is being studied further.

A HER2/neu peptide (a small part of the protein produced by the HER2/neu gene), used as the antigen in an antigen vaccine, has been shown to cause an increased immune response against the HER2/neu receptor; it is under continuing study.

Other specific antigen vaccines have also shown promise and are being developed. These vaccines are almost always used after primary therapy (lumpectomy and radiation therapy, or mastectomy) and sometimes together with hormonal therapy or chemotherapy, to try to prevent the cancer from coming back.

## Biological therapy

Is a treatment designed to enhance the body's natural defenses by stimulating or restoring ability of immune system to fight infection and disease. It is known as immunotherapy.

## Gene therapy

One gene that has been implicated in various cancers is the p53 gene. This gene makes protein that is responsible for stopping uncontrolled growth of a cell. A vaccine containing very high level of this p53 protein is injected into or near the site of cancer .It has the ability to make cancer cells more sensitive to the killing effect of chemotherapy.

## Targeted Therapies

A targeted therapy is one that is designed to treat only the cancer cells and minimize damage to normal, healthy cells. Cancer treatments that 'target' cancer cells may offer the advantage of reduced treatment-related side effects and improved outcomes.

Conventional cancer treatments, such as chemotherapy and radiation therapy, cannot distinguish between cancer cells and healthy cells. Consequently, healthy cells are commonly damaged in the process of treating the cancer, which results in side effects. Chemotherapy damages rapidly dividing cells, a hallmark trait of cancer cells. In the process, healthy cells that are also rapidly dividing, such as blood cells and the cells lining the mouth and gastro intestinal tract are also damaged. Radiation therapy kills some healthy cells that are in the path of the radiation or near the cancer being treated. Newer radiation therapy techniques can reduce, but not eliminate this damage. Treatment-related damage to healthy cells leads to complications of treatment, or side effects. These side effects may be severe, reducing a patient's quality of life, compromising their ability to receive their full, prescribed treatment, and sometimes, limiting their chance for an optimal outcome from treatment.

Chapter 12

# Side Effects of Treatment of Breast Cancer

## Chemotherapy[95]

Chemotherapy does not only target cancer cells, but any cells that divide rapidly. This includes those in the bone marrow and skin, hair-producing cells, and the cells that line the mouth and digestive system. Damage to these healthy cells may produce various side effects, including:

- Tiredness
- Nausea and vomiting
- Diarrhea or constipation
- Hair loss
- Getting infections more easily
- Sore mouth, mouth ulcers and changes in the sense of taste

Many of these side-effects can be controlled using additional drugs. For example, nausea can be reduced using antemetic (anti-sickness) drugs such as ondansetron or steroids (eg dexamethasone). Furthermore, most side-effects are temporary and will pass once treatment is completed. However, there is a risk that irreversible infertility and, for women, early menopause may occur.

## Effects on everyday life

Some people manage to continue with their lives normally during chemotherapy. A small number of people even feel better as the symptoms of their cancer decrease. However, for many people, chemotherapy can have significant effects on everyday life. In particular, tiredness often prevents patients from carrying on working full time or doing normal levels of physical activity.

Women having chemotherapy should not try to become pregnant during treatment because the chemotherapy drugs can damage the developing baby.

## Surgery

In the past, most breast cancer surgeries involved the removal of the breast (mastectomy). More recently, however, many women have been given the option of breast-conserving surgery or lumpectomy with radiation therapy. Clinical trials have proven that both options provide the same long-term survival rates for most types of early breast cancer.

With lumpectomy, the surgeon removes the breast cancer and some normal tissue around it in order to achieve 'clean margins.' A 'clean margin' is achieved when tissue on the outer edge of the surgery has no evidence of the disease. Usually, the surgeon also takes out some of the lymph nodes under the arm to find out if the cancer has spread.

Lumpectomy is often followed by radiation therapy to destroy any cancer cells that may not have been removed or detected at the time of surgery.

Depending on the size and location of the cancer, mastectomy may be recommended. This entails removal of most or all of the breast, possibly including the lining over the chest muscles and sometimes part of the chest wall muscles. Some of the lymph nodes under the arm are also taken out to check for spread of the cancer.

Mastectomy is sometimes followed by radiation therapy,

depending upon the size of the tumor and if any lymph nodes have cancer - to destroy any cancer cells that may not have been removed or detectable at the time of surgery.

Breast reconstruction is often an option after mastectomy. This may involve the use of a flap of skin, muscle and fat from another part of the body to create a breast shape. An implant (saline or silicone-filled sac) may also be used to form a breast mound. Reconstruction can be done at the same time as mastectomy in some cases thus avoiding a second operation. Also, a sentinel node biopsy can be an option instead of traditional lymph node removal under the arm. This entails injecting a dye or radioactive tracer into the tumor bed and removing the lymph node that absorbs it first (the sentinel node). This procedure has fewer side effects and is very effective in experienced hands.

## Lymphedema

The lymphatic system helps coordinate the immune system's function to protect the body from foreign substances and includes an extensive network of lymph vessels and lymph nodes. Here's how the lymphatic system works:

- Excess fluid is collected from the space between tissues in the body and moves through the lymph vessels. The fluid (now called lymph) isn't pumped through the body like blood, but instead is 'pushed' through the lymph system as the vessels are compressed by surrounding muscles.
- Filters called lymph nodes remove certain harmful substances from the lymph fluid, such as bacteria and debris. The fluid from most tissues or organs is filtered through one or more lymph nodes before draining into the bloodstream.

### What is Lymphedema?[96]

Lymphedema is an abnormal buildup of fluid that causes swelling, most often in the arms or legs. The condition develops when lymph vessels or lymph nodes are missing, impaired, damaged or removed.

There are two types of lymphedema: primary and secondary.

Primary lymphedema is rare and is caused by the absence of, or abnormalities in, certain lymph vessels at birth.

Secondary lymphedema occurs as a result of a blockage or interruption that alters the flow of lymph through the lymphatic system and can develop from an infection, malignancy, surgery, scar tissue formation, trauma, deep vein thrombosis (blood clot in a vein), radiation, or other cancer treatment.

## Who is at risk for developing Lymphedema?

People who have had any of the following procedures may be at risk for developing lymphedema:

- Simple mastectomy in combination with axillary (armpit) lymph node removal
- Lumpectomy in combination with axillary lymph node removal
- Modified radical mastectomy in combination with axillary lymph node removal
- Combined cancer surgery and radiation therapy to a lymph node region (such as the neck, armpit, groin, pelvis or abdomen)
- Radiation therapy to a lymph node region

Lymphedema can occur within a few days, months, or years after surgery. A small amount of swelling is normal for the first four to six weeks after surgery.

## What happens after breast surgery?

Lymphedema develops after breast surgery because there is an alteration in the pathway that drains the fluids involved in the immune system. It can occur at any time after the surgery. If untreated, it can become worse.

Following surgery, a physician will examine you and take arm measurements. Sometimes, there may be redness or pain in the arm, which may be a sign of inflammation. Depending on your symptoms, your physician will then consider the best treatment options for you.

## What are the signs and symptoms of Lymphedema?

If you suspect any of the symptoms listed below, call your healthcare provider right away. Prompt treatment can help get the condition under control.

- Swelling in the arms, hands, fingers, shoulders, chest or legs. The swelling may occur for the first time after a traumatic event (such as bruises, cuts, sunburn, and sports injuries), after an infection in the part of the body that was treated for cancer, or after an extended (more than three hours) airplane trip (due to the sudden change in cabin pressure).
- A 'full' or heavy sensation in the arms or legs
- Skin tightness
- Decreased flexibility in the hand, wrist or ankle
- Difficulty fitting into clothing in one specific area
- Tight-fitting bracelet, watch or ring that wasn't tight before

## How is Lymphedema diagnosed?

Lymphedema is diagnosed after a careful evaluation of your medical history, including past surgeries and treatments, an evaluation of current medications and symptoms, and a complete physical examination. Sometimes, additional tests may be needed.

## How is Lymphedema treated?

Lymphedema treatments vary, depending on the stage and cause of the illness. The most important aspect of treatment is learning how to care for your health. Your doctor or nurse will teach you and your family how to follow your prescribed treatment.

If the initial signs and symptoms of swelling are caused by infection, antibiotics may be prescribed. Other treatments may include bandaging, proper skin care and diet, compression garments, exercises and manual lymphatic drainage, a gentle form of skin stretching/massage.

## How can I help prevent Lymphedema?

Lymphedema can be prevented or controlled (if it develops) by following the recommendations below.

### Maintain good nutrition

- Reduce foods high in salt and fat
- Include at least two to four servings of fruits and three to five servings of vegetables in your daily meal plan
- Eat a variety of foods to get all the nutrients you need
- Use the package label information to help you to make the best selections for a healthy lifestyle
- Eat foods high in fiber such as whole-grain breads, cereals, pasta, rice, fresh fruits and vegetables
- Drink plenty of water, eight ounce glasses of water per day
- Maintain your ideal body weight. (A registered dietician or your health-care provider can help calculate your ideal body weight.)
- Avoid alcoholic beverages

### Exercise regularly

- Always check with your physician first before starting a new exercise program.
- To improve cardiovascular fitness, you should perform aerobic activities (including walking, swimming, low-impact aerobics or specially prescribed exercises) for twenty to thirty minutes at least three times a week.
- Take time to include a five-minute warm-up, including stretching exercises, before any aerobic activity and include a five to ten-minutes cool down after the activity.
- If your normal exercise routine includes weight lifting with your arms, check with your doctor about the best time to resume this activity and if there are any weight restrictions.
- Discontinue any exercise that causes unexpected pain. If your arm or leg (on the side where you had surgery) becomes tired during exercise, cool down, then rest and elevate it.

## Avoid infections

- Wear gloves while doing housework or gardening.
- Avoid cutting your cuticles when manicuring your nails. Take care when cutting your toenails.
- Frequently wash your hands with soap and warm water, especially before preparing food, and after using the bathroom or after touching soiled linens or clothes.
- Protect your skin from scratches, sores, burns and other irritations that might lead to infection. Use electric razors to remove hair and replace the razor top frequently.
- Use insect repellents to prevent bug bites.
- Immediately report any signs of infection to your physician.

## Stay alert for signs of infection

- Fever over 100 degrees F (38 degrees C)
- Sweats or chills
- Skin rash
- Pain, tenderness, redness or swelling
- Wound or cut that won't heal
- Red, warm or draining sore
- Sore throat, scratchy throat or pain when swallowing
- Sinus drainage, nasal congestion, headaches or tenderness along upper cheekbones
- Persistent dry or moist cough that lasts more than two days
- White patches in your mouth or on your tongue
- Nausea, vomiting or diarrhea
- Flu-like symptoms (chills, aches, headache or fatigue) or generally feeling 'lousy'
- Trouble urinating, pain or burning, constant urge or frequent urination
- Bloody, cloudy or foul-smelling urine

## Avoid tight clothing, shoes or jewelry

Women should wear well-fitted bras; bra straps should not be too tight, avoid underwire styles, and wear pads under the bra straps if necessary. Wear comfortable, closed-toe shoes and avoid tight hosiery. Wear watches or jewelery loosely, if at all, on the affected arm (surgical side).

## Avoid heavy lifting with the affected arm (even a purse or bag)

Avoid repetitive movements of the affected arm (such as scrubbing, pushing or pulling). Do not carry a purse or bag on your shoulder (the side where you had surgery).

## Keep your skin meticulously clean

Dry your skin thoroughly (including creases and between fingers and toes) and apply lotion.

## Take precautions during visits to your doctor

Ask to have your blood pressure checked on the unaffected arm (nonsurgical side) and avoid injections or blood drawing on the surgical side if possible.

## Inform your doctor of any symptoms

Notify your doctor if you have redness, swelling, a skin rash or blister on the side of your body where you had surgery, or if you have a temperature over 100 degrees F (38 degrees C). These warning signs of infection could be an early sign of lymphedema and should be treated immediately.

## What can you do if you already have Lymphedema?

To help decrease the risk of further swelling, continue following the recommendations for preventing lymphedema listed above. In addition:

- Avoid extreme temperature changes. Do not use hot tubs, whirlpools, saunas or steam baths. Use warm, rather than very

hot, water when bathing or washing dishes. Always wear sun protection (at least SPF 15) when going outdoors.
- When traveling by air, ask your healthcare provider if you should wear a compression sleeve on your affected arm or a stocking on your affected leg. For long flights, additional bandages may be needed. Talk to your healthcare provider before traveling.
- When sitting or sleeping, elevate your affected arm or leg on pillows. Avoid prolonged lying on your affected side.
- Your physician may refer you to an occupational therapist who specializes in managing lymphedema. The therapist will assess your condition and develop an individual treatment plan to manage your lymphedema.
- Therapy may include specific exercises or a complete exercise program, limitation of certain activities that are vigorous or repetitive, and recommendations for a compression sleeve, bandages, manual lymph drainage and possibly a pump.
- Continue to see your health-care provider for frequent follow-up visits, as recommended.

## What is the outlook?

Lymphedema cannot be cured. However, with proper care and treatment, the affected limb can be restored to a normal size and shape. In addition, lymphedema can be treated and controlled so that it does not progress further.

If left untreated, lymphedema can lead to increased swelling and a hardening of the tissue, resulting in decreased function and mobility in the affected limb. It can also lead to chronic infections and other illnesses.

It is important to receive treatment promptly if you recognize symptoms of lymphedema.

After surgery you will have a dressing (bandage) over the surgery site. You may have one or more drains (plastic or rubber tubes) from the breast or underarm area to remove blood and lymph fluid that collects during the healing process. Care of the drains includes emptying and measuring the fluid and identifying problems the doctor or nurse needs to know about. Most drains stay in place for one or two weeks.

Doctors rarely put the arm in a sling to hold it in place. Most doctors will want you to start moving the arm so that it won't get stiff. Women who have a lumpectomy or mastectomy are surprised by how little pain they have in the breast area. But they are less happy with the strange sensations (numbness, pinching/pulling feeling) in the underarm area.

Written instructions about care after surgery should be given to the patient and their caregivers. These instructions should include:

- The care of the surgical wound and dressing
- How to monitor drainage and take care of the drains
- How to recognize signs of infection
- When to call the doctor or nurse
- When to begin using the arm and how to do arm exercises to prevent stiffness
- When to resume wearing a bra
- When to begin using a prosthesis and what type to use (after mastectomy)
- What to eat and not to eat
- Use of medications, including pain medicines
- Any restrictions of activity
- What to expect regarding sensations or numbness in the breast and arm
- What to expect regarding feelings about body image
- A follow-up appointment and referral to a breast cancer recovery volunteer. A volunteer who has had breast cancer can provide information, comfort, and support.

Most patients see their doctor within seven to fourteen days following the surgery. Your doctor should explain the results of your pathology report and talk to you about the need for further treatment. If you will need more treatment, you will be referred to a medical oncologist and/or radiation oncologist.

## Radiation therapy

Side effects depend mainly on the dose and type of radiation and the part of your body that is being treated.

It is common for the skin in the treated area to become red, dry, tender, and itchy. Your breast may feel heavy and tight. These problems will go away over time. Toward the end of treatment, your skin may become moist and 'weepy'. Exposing this area to air as much as possible can help the skin heal.

Bras and some other types of clothing may rub your skin and cause soreness. You may want to wear loose-fitting cotton clothes during this time. Gentle skin care also is important. You should check with your doctor before using any deodorants, lotions, or creams on the treated area. These effects of radiation therapy on the skin will go away. The area gradually heals once treatment is over. However, there may be a lasting change in the colour of your skin.

You are likely to become very tired during radiation therapy, especially in the later weeks of treatment. Resting is important, but doctors usually advise patients to try to stay as active as they can.

Although the side effects of radiation therapy can be distressing, your doctor can usually relieve them.

You may want to ask your doctor these questions before having radiation therapy:

- How will radiation be given?
- When will the treatment start? When will it end? How often will I have treatments?
- How will I feel during treatment? Will I be able to drive myself to and from the treatment?
- How will we know the treatment is working?
- What can I do to take care of myself before, during, and after the treatment?

- Will the treatment affect my skin?
- How will my chest look afterward
- Are there any long-term effects?
- What is the chance that the cancer will come back in my breast?

Please remember that the extent and the exact type of side effects are determined by the location of the tumor and the location of the radiation being delivered. Patients should check with their radiation oncologists in advance so that they are warned of any of these potential side effects.

For instance, patients who are undergoing breast irradiation will typically experience a redness, dryness or itchiness of the breasts that usually begins two to three weeks after the treatment is commenced. It will then continue, but will eventually leave several weeks after the radiation treatment course is completed.

Other examples are diarrhea, nausea or vomiting. This is sometimes experienced by patients undergoing radiation treatment to their abdomens or bowels. In most cases, these side effects, which are called acute, take place during the radiation treatment course and will continue for a few weeks after the course is completed.

In almost all cases, these side effects will go away and the patients will be fine. In rare instances, some patients will experience long-term side effects or complications, because the radiation causes damage to an internal organ adjacent to or near the tumor site.

Radiation can sometimes play a role in the development of cancer, particularly if people are exposed to it at an early age. We are all aware of the increased frequency of cancers, especially Leukemias, among Japanese survivors of World War II. Patients should bear in mind that radiation, as delivered in a radiation department, is a very careful, precise and well monitored treatment which very rarely leads to the development of cancer.

Radiation therapy targets specific areas where cancer cells have formed tumors. However, it can also affect healthy cells in the immediate vicinity. As a result, some side-effects may occur. The most common include:

- **Skin damage:** The skin in the treated area may be somewhat sensitive and therefore should be protected against exposure to sunlight and irritation. Besides feeling tender, the skin often will become red and irritated. However, actual burns are rare with modern radiotherapy techniques. Also, your physician may prescribe an antibiotic ointment, or steroid cream to relieve itching and pain and to speed healing in severe cases of skin breakdown.
- **Hair loss:** Hair is frequently lost from the area receiving the radiation therapy. However, the hair will sometimes grow back once the treatment is finished.
- **Nausea, vomiting and headaches:** These side effects can occur following radiation therapy to specific sites, such as the head or abdomen. They can often be relieved and sometimes prevented by certain medications. Radiation to the breast or chest wall rarely causes any nausea.

Other side effects may occur depending on the specific area being treated.

## Hormone therapy

Some breast tumors need hormones to grow. Hormone therapy keeps cancer cells from getting or using the natural hormones they need. These hormones are estrogen and progesterone. Laboratory tests can show if a breast tumor has hormone receptors. If you have this kind of tumor, you may have hormone therapy.

This treatment uses drugs or surgery.

**Drugs:** Your doctor may suggest a drug that can block the natural hormone. One drug is tamoxifen, which blocks estrogen. Another type of drug prevents the body from making the female hormone estradiol. Estradiol is a form of estrogen. This type of drug is an aromatase inhibitor. If you have not gone through menopause, your doctor may give you a drug that stops the ovaries from making estrogen.

**Surgery:** If you have not gone through menopause, you may have surgery to remove your ovaries. The ovaries are the main source of the body's estrogen. A woman who has gone through menopause does not need surgery. (The ovaries produce less estrogen after menopause.)

The side effects of hormone therapy depend largely on the specific drug or type of treatment. Tamoxifen is the most common hormone treatment. In general, the side effects of tamoxifen are similar to some of the symptoms of menopause. The most common are hot flushes and vaginal discharges. Other side effects are irregular menstrual periods, headaches, fatigue, nausea, vomiting, vaginal dryness or itching, irritation of the skin around the vagina, and skin rash. Not all women who take tamoxifen have side effects.

It is possible to become pregnant when taking tamoxifen, but it migth harm the unborn baby. If you are still menstruating, you should discuss birth control methods with your doctor.

Serious side effects of tamoxifen are rare. However, it can cause blood clots in the veins. Blood clots form most often in the legs and in the lungs. Women have a slight increase in their risk of stroke.

Tamoxifen can cause cancer of the uterus. Your doctor should perform regular pelvic exams. You should tell your doctor about any unusual vaginal bleeding between examinations.

When the ovaries are removed, menopause occurs at once. The side effects are often more severe than those caused by natural menopause. Your health care provider can suggest ways to cope with these side effects.

If laboratory tests show that a tumor depends on your natural hormones to grow, it will be described as estrogen-positive or progesterone-positive in the laboratory report. This means that any remaining cancer cell may continue to grow when these hormones are present in your body. Hormonal therapy can block your body's natural hormones from reaching any remaining cancer cell.

One of the most common hormonal therapies is tamoxifen, which has been used for nearly twenty years to treat patients with advanced stage breast cancer. Now it is also being used as additional treatment for early stage disease to prevent recurrence and recent clinical trials have even shown it to be effective in preventing breast cancer in people at high risk for the future development of breast cancer.

Possible side effects from hormonal therapy may include hot flushes, nausea, menstrual irregularities or changes in fertility such as an increased incidence of spontaneous abortion. Often these disappear after treatment ends. The side effects of most concern from tamoxifen are an increased risk of developing uterine cancer and blood clots. These risks are small and usually the benefit from tamoxifen outweighs the risks, but a thorough discussion with the doctor is imperative.

Many other hormonal therapies exist and new drugs are in development. Hormonal therapy is a very important way to treat breast and it is now recognized that it benefits more groups of patients.

## Biological therapy

Biological therapy helps the immune system fight cancer. The immune system is the body's natural defense against disease.

Some women with breast cancer, that has spread, receive a biological therapy called Herceptin® (trastuzumab). It is a monoclonal antibody. It is made in the laboratory and binds to cancer cells.

Herceptin is given to women whose laboratory tests show that a breast tumor has too much of a specific protein known as HER2, by blocking this protein it can slow or stop the growth of the cancer cells.

Herceptin is given by vein. It may be given alone or with chemotherapy.

The first time a woman receives Herceptin, the most common side effects are fever and chills. Some women also have pain, weakness, nausea, vomiting, diarrhea, headaches, difficulty breathing, or rashes. Side effects usually become milder after the first treatment.

Herceptin also may cause heart damage. This may lead to heart failure. Herceptin can also affect the lungs. It can cause breathing problems that require a doctor at once. Before you receive Herceptin, your doctor will check for your heart and lungs. During treatment, your doctor will watch for signs of lung problems.

Chapter 13

# Evidence Based Management of Patients

## Guidelines

Since breast cancer treatment depends on a number of factors and it can create confusion as to which type of treatment modality to follow, evidence based management guidelines for management of breast cancer patients have been compiled by the Tata Memorial Cancer Hospital, Mumbai.[97]

Patients are clinically grouped into one of the following categories:

- Operable Breast Cancer
- Large Operable Breast Cancer
- Locally Advanced Breast Cancer
- Metastatic Breast Cancer

## Criteria

Operable Breast Cancer:
- T< 5cm, N0 or N1 mobile, M0

Large Operable Breast Cancer:
- T> 5cm with no skin involvement, N0 or N1, M0

Locally Advanced Breast Cancer:
i.  Skin involvement in the form of edema, ulceration, infiltration, satellite nodules
ii. Matted or fixed axillary lymph nodes
iii. Ipsilateral supraclavicular/internal mammary lymph node(s)
iv. Fixity to chest wall
v.  Arm edema
vi. No evidence of distant metastasis

## Operable Breast Cancer

Clinical Examination and Investigations:
i.  Documentation of exact extent of primary tumor and axillary node(s)
ii. Pathological confirmation of diagnosis by FNAC/ Incision biopsy
iii. Bilateral film mammogram (mandatory if BCT is contemplated)
iv. Routine pre-anesthetic tests including chest X-ray and LFT
v.  ER / PgR if neoadjuvant chemotherapy is planned

**Note:** A strong clinical suspicion for malignancy over-rules both negative FNAC or mammography for excision biopsy

**Metastatic work up:** Is not recommended routinely in operable breast cancer, as the incidence of metastasis is <2%. These tests have a low sensitivity and are not cost-effective.

## Surgical Options

i.  Breast Conservative Therapy (BCT)-Wide excision with complete axillary clearance up to apex.
ii. Modified Radical Mastectomy (MRM).

**NB:** Sentinel node biopsy is presently an investigational procedure

Contraindications to BCT:
- Multicentric disease (> 1 quadrant)
- Extensive microcalcification on mammogram
- Doubtful compliance with adjuvant radiotherapy
- Pregnancy (first/second trimesters and previous child)
- Satisfactory cosmesis unlikely (relative contraindication)

Options for BCT for relatively large tumors:
- Down-staging with neo-adjuvant Chemotherapy
- BCT with latissimus dorsi reconstruction

Model Histopathology Report
- Tumor size (all 3 dimensions)
- Tumor type
- Tumor grade (Modified Richardson Bloom Score)
- Presence of extensive intraductal carcinoma (EIC)*
- Lymphovascular embolisation
- Cut Margin status (gross positive/ focal positive/ negative) in case of lumpectomy or wide excision**
- Number of positive/total axillary lymph node dissected
- Receptor status: ER and PgR (by IHC or EIA)

**Note:**
* EIC is defined as presence of DCIS in more than 25 percent of any low power field within or outside the tumor and is a strong predictor of local recurrence after BCT.
** Gross +ve cut margin is extensive involvement of a cut margin or more than 3 foci of invasive or in-situ carcinoma in any inked margin (requires revision excision or mastectomy).
** Focal positive cut margin is three or less foci of invasive or in-situ carcinoma in any inked margin (Revision surgery only if EIC positive).

## Adjuvant Therapy

**Modalities**

Systemic: Hormone-therapy and or Polychemotherapy Locoregional: Radiotherapy Candidates for Adjuvant Systemic Therapy: All women with node-positive breast cancer and / or >1 cm tumor ER or PgR + ve ER and PgR -ve Premenopausal Chemotherapy + Hormonal therapy Chemotherapy only Postmenopausal Hormonal therapy +/- Chemotherapy Hormonal therapy + Chemotherapy Ovarian ablation considered in pre-menopausal women > 40 years with ER positive tumour. In postmenopausal women with ER positive tumor, Tamoxifen or Anastrozole can be used. Doses and schedules of adjuvant systemic therapy

i. Adjuvant Hormone therapy
- Tamoxifen: 20 mg/day for a period of 5 years
- Anastrazole: 2.5 mg / day for a period of 5 years

ii. Adjuvant Polychemotherapy (IV bolus or infusion)

CAF: D1 only at 3 weekly intervals x 6 cycles

Cyclophosphamide 600 mg/m$^2$

Adriamycin 60 mg/m$^2$

5-fluorouracil 600 mg/m$^2$

CEF: D1 only at 3 weekly intervals x 6 cycles

Cyclophosphamide 500 mg/m$^2$

Epirubicin 90 mg/m$^2$

5-fluorouracil 500 mg/m$^2$

AC: D1 only at 3 weekly intervals x 4 cycles

Cyclophosphamide 600 mg/m$^2$

Adriamycin 60 mg/m$^2$

CMF: D1 and D8 at monthly intervals x 6 cycles

Cyclophosphamide 600 mg/m$^2$

Methotrexate 40 mg/m$^2$

5-fluorouracil 600 mg/m$^2$

## Candidates for adjuvant loco-regional radio-therapy

i. Breast conservation surgery: All patients should receive radiotherapy.

ii. Post MRM: T >5cm, skin/chest wall involvement or axillary node metastases. In the absence of other risk factors, locoregional RT may be avoided for <4 metastatic axillary nodes if the axillary surgery was adequate.

iii. For women who receive post operative RT, the radiation target volume includes breast / chest wall in all cases and SCF nodes when >3 axillary nodes are +ve.

**Dose recommended:** equivalent to 45 to 50 Gy / 25# / 5 wks. Tumor bed boost with electrons or 192 Iridium implant (LDR or HDR), equivalent to 10-15 Gy is recommended for all BCTs.

Routine post operative irradiation of axilla is not recommended unless there is known or suspected residual axillary disease. Similarly, routine irradiation of internal mammary nodes is not recommended pending the results of the large EORTC trial examining the survival benefit of internal mammary RT possible cardiac morbidity / mortality with IMC irradiation.

## Locally Advanced Breast Cancer

Investigations

i. Incision Biopsy for tissue diagnosis and receptor study
ii. Mammography or breast sonography for baseline documentation of tumor size
iii. Following metastatic work-up is recommended
- Chest radiography
- Ultrasound abdomen
- Liver function test
- Radionuclide Bone Scan
- Relevant skeletal X-rays

## Treatment plan multi-modal therapy

- Sequence Neo-adjuvant chemotherapy followed by surgery followed by completion chemotherapy and then locoregional RT (plus tamoxifen if ER +ve).
- Neo-adjuvant Chemotherapy with CAF / CEF
  Dose schedules are same as for adjuvant chemotherapy.

  Clinical documentation of response at each cycle (primary tumor and nodal size) till maximum tumor shrinkage is achieved (i.e. measurements at two consecutive CT cycles is constant) or there is clinical progression (usually 2 - 6 cycles).

## Surgical treatment options

i. If clinical and radiological (mammography) complete response index quadrantectomy with axillary clearance (BCT).

ii. If partial response with radiological evidence of residual disease (a) BCT where feasible or (b) SMAC.

iii. If static disease or progressive disease SMAC with or without reconstruction for skin cover so that post-operative radiation can be instituted early.

iv. In case of disease progression locally with inoperability of disease may consider for preoperative radiotherapy followed by reassessment for surgical excision later.

**Completion of remaining cycles of chemotherapy:** (Total 6 cycles) However, if there was no response or disease progression during pre-operative chemotherapy, post operative RT is given first followed by consideration of second line chemotherapy.

Tamoxifen (if ER / PR +ve) for a period of five years.

**Postoperative Radiotherapy:** All patients with LABC should receive RT to the breast or chest wall to a dose equivalent of 50 Gy/ 25# / 5 wks (or 45 Gy / 20# / 4 wks). If BCT has been performed a tumor bed boost of 15 Gy in six fractions with appropriate electrons is recommended. Routine postoperative irradiation of axilla is not recommended unless there is known or suspected residual axillary disease. Similarly, routine irradiation of internal mammary nodes is not recommended pending the results of the large EORTC trial examining the survival benefit of internal mammary RT possible cardiac morbidity / mortality with IMC irradiation is awaited.

## Follow-up after primary treatment of breast cancer

i. Bi-annual Physical Examination (PE) for five years followed by yearly checkup
ii. Mammography once in eighteen months
iii. No other investigations in asymptomatic patients for early detection of metastasis, since it is -
    - Not cost-effective
    - Does not prolong survival
    - Detection and disclosure of spread of disease may be psychologically harmful to an asymptomatic patient with an incurable metastatic disease.

If recurrence or symptoms suggestive of metastasis, relevant investigations to be done are:

- Chest radiography
- Ultrasound abdomen
- Liver function test
- Radionuclide bone scan
- Skeletal survey of suspicious or weight bearing areas
- CT / MRI, where indicated

## Treatment of isolated loco-regional recurrence

Resectable: Surgery + radiotherapy

On completion of loco-regional treatment if there is no evaluable disease then, tamoxifen (for ER or PgR +ve tumor) till progression. There is no evidence that early institution of chemotherapy (in ER -ve tumors) prolongs survival, hence it is not recommended.

Unresectable or within the field of previous radiotherapy:
- Chemotherapy followed by assessment for surgery
- Metastatic Breast Cancer
- Goal of management is palliation

Options and Principles of Management
- Hormone therapy
- Chemotherapy
- Radiotherapy
- Surgery: Pleurodesis, Palliative mastectomy

Spinal decompression
- Analgesics, Anti-emetics, Sedatives
- Others: Bisphosphonates

# Nerve blocks

Decision to use chemotherapy or hormone therapy is based on receptor status, disease-free interval (DFI), tempo of recurrent disease and the site of metastasis (whether life-threatening).

## Hormone therapy

For ER or PgR +ve; exclusive bone and soft tissue metastasis, slow tempo of disease or DFI>1 year:

First line: Tamoxifen (20 mg) / Letrozole (2.5mg)

Second/Third line: Letrozole (2.5mg) / Exemestane (25mg) Medroxy-progesterone acetate (100 mg tid), Megesterol acetate (40 mg qid)

Oophorectomy - in premenopausal ER and /or PgR positive women as second line of treatment.

## Chemotherapy

For ER and PR -ve disease, visceral metastasis, fast tempo of disease or DFI<1 year:

First line CAF / CEF

Second line   Paclitaxel (3 wkly 135mg infusion over 3hrs), Docetaxel (3 wkly 100mg infusion over 3hrs)

Taxanes + carboplatin or adriamycin

Mitomycin + Mitoxantrone + Methotrexate

(Doses: Mitomycin and Mitoxantrone 10mg/m$^2$ Methotrexate 40 mg/m$^2$ )

Third line CMF

## Radiation therapy

**Bone metastases:** For pain relief, preventing or treating neurological and skeletal complications of bone metastases.

**Isolated or few bone metastases:** Localized RT to a dose of 8 Gy single fraction or 20 Gy/5#/1wk, if there is a risk of pathological fracture or impending / established cord compression.

**Widespread bone metastases:** Hemi Body Irradiation (HBI); Upper HBI 6 Gy / 1#; Lower HBI 8 Gy/1#. When both halves of the body have to be treated there should be an interval of 6 weeks.

**Brain metastasis:** For relieving / preventing neurological manifestation of brain metastases

**Solitary brain metastases (extracranial disease controlled) and good performance status:** Whole brain RT (30 Gy/10#/2wks). Whenever feasible, consider surgical excision prior to whole brain RT or Radiosurgery boost after whole brain RT.

**Multiple brain mets or uncontrolled extracranial disease or poor performance status:** Whole brain RT (20 Gy/5#/1wk or 12 Gy/2#/3 days).

**Choroidal metastases:** Palliative RT (20 Gy/5# or 30 Gy/10#)

## Bisphosphonates

**Lytic bone metastasis in weight bearing areas:** Pamidronate I.V 90mg, 4 weekly (or other bisphosphonates) as an adjuvant to RT for prevention of fractures and pain relief.

## Prognosis

The best indicators of the course of the disease and its outcome in breast cancer are the tumor size and lymph node involvement. Prognosis depends not on the duration for which the tumor has been present but on its invasiveness and metastatic potential. In attempt to define which tumor will behave aggressively and require early systematic treatment, a host of prognostic factors have been described like hormone receptor status, histological grading of tumor, oncogene and growth factor analysis.

Chapter 14

# Issues after Breast Cancer Treatment

## Follow Up[98]

After the first course of treatment is completed, it is very important to go to all scheduled follow-up appointments. During these appointments, your doctors will ask questions about any symptoms, do physical examinations, and order laboratory or imaging tests as needed to find recurrences or side effects. You should never hesitate to tell your doctor or other members of your cancer care team about any symptoms or side effects that concern you.

At first, your follow-up appointments will probably be scheduled for every four to six months. The longer you have been free of cancer, the less often the appointments are needed. After five years, they are done once a year. You will need to have yearly mammograms of the remaining breast and the breast treated by lumpectomy.

If you are taking tamoxifen, you should have yearly pelvic examinations because this drug can increase your risk of uterine cancer. Be sure to tell your doctor right away about any abnormal vaginal bleeding you are having. Although excessive or irregular vaginal bleeding is usually caused by a non-cancerous condition, it may also be the first sign of uterine cancer.

If you are taking an aromatase inhibitor, you should consider testing your bone density.

Other tests such as blood tumor marker studies, blood tests of liver function, bone scans, and chest x-rays are not usually needed unless symptoms or physical examination findings suggest it is likely that the cancer has recurred. These and other tests may be done as part of evaluating new treatments by clinical trials.

If initial examinations and tests suggest a recurrence, a chest x-ray, CT scan, PET scan, MRI scan, bone scan, and/or a biopsy may be done. Your doctor may also measure the tumor marker CA-15-3, CA 27-29, or CEA with a blood test. The blood level of these substance goes up in some women if their cancer has spread to bones or other organs such as the liver. Depending on the location of a recurrent cancer, treatment may involve surgery, radiation therapy, hormone therapy, and/or chemotherapy.

## Lymphedema

Lymphedema, or swelling of the arm due to buildup of fluid, may occur after the treatment of breast cancer. Any treatment that involves axillary dissection or radiation to the axillary lymph nodes carries the risk of lymphedema because normal drainage of lymph from the arm is disrupted.

The onset of lymphedema is often subtle and unpredictable. There is no good way to predict who will and will not develop lymphedema. It can occur right after surgery, or months or even years later. The potential for developing lymphedema remains throughout a woman's lifetime.

With care, lymphedema can often be avoided or, if it develops, kept under control. Injury or infection involving the affected arm or hand can contribute to the development of lymphedema or aggravate existing lymphedema, so preventive measures should focus on protecting the arm and hand. Most doctors recommend that women avoid having blood drawn from the arm that has lymphedema.

One of the first symptoms of lymphedema may be a feeling of tightness in the arm or hand on the same side that was treated for breast cancer. Any swelling, tightness, or injury to the arm or hand should be reported promptly to your doctor or nurse. Pressure garments is also suggested to decrease the lymphedema.

## Pregnancy after Breast Cancer [99,100]

Less than 10 percent of women who have been treated for breast cancer will desire a future pregnancy. Therefore, the amount of data that is available to answer this question is relatively small. Appreciating this limitation, the existing data has demonstrated that, after adjusting for age, stage of disease, and reproductive history prior to breast cancer treatment, women who have a post therapy full term pregnancy have no significant difference in their cancer-outcome than do women who do not become pregnant. An important consideration, however, is what difference would it make to the woman if she knew that her cancer was going to return? Would she opt not to become pregnant, choosing to avoid bringing a child into the world, a child that has a high chance of losing its biologic mother ? Or would the patient choose to reproduce so that a legacy could be established ? These are all difficult questions, the answers to which are highly personal. Many medical oncologists will attempt to minimize the necessity to even answer these questions by encouraging women to delay child bearing for about two years after the completion of the first treatment for breast cancer. The rationale for this tact is based upon the realization that the majority of young women who do develop recurrent breast cancer will do such within the first two years. By delaying reproduction beyond this time window, the probability that a patient is going to have to make these difficult decisions is decreased, though not eliminated.

A number of women who have successfully undergone treatment for breast cancer wish to have further pregnancies. Stage for stage, breast cancer during pregnancy has a similar prognosis (outcome) to that of breast cancer in young, non-pregnant women. According to recent studies, women who have been successfully treated for breast cancer in the past do not usually experience fertility problems unless chemotherapy is administered as part of the treatment. Premenopausal women treated with chemotherapy should be aware that the treatment can cause infertility and/or premature menopause, especially in older pre-menopausal woman (typically in their forties) who are already naturally less fertile and closer to menopause.

For women diagnosed with early-stage breast cancer, pregnancy is usually reasonable two or more years after diagnosis and treatment. However, some women may be advised to have children sooner if they are older and there are other considerations. Several details such as cancer type, degree of metastasis (spread) and amount of radiation and/or chemotherapy received should be considered before advising a woman whether it is safe to become pregnant after breast cancer. For example, those at higher risk of an early recurrence may be advised to wait and be closely observed prior to attempting a pregnancy. If a pregnancy is successful after having been treated for breast cancer, some women who have had radiation therapy on one breast find that a sufficient amount of milk for breast-feeding cannot be produced by the irradiated (treated) breast. However, the other, normal breast can often produce enough milk to enable breast-feeding.

Women with Stage IV (metastatic) breast cancer or recurrent tumors may not be good candidates for future pregnancies. Chemotherapy may also have an adverse effect on the ovaries and lead to fertility problems or a higher rate of spontaneous miscarriages. However, each individual is different, and all pre-menopausal women should discuss the issue of future pregnancies with their physicians before their initial breast cancer treatment, if they are interested in having children after treatment. In some cases, women may wish to consider banking eggs prior to treatment (particularly chemotherapy) if they wish to have children in the future. Women taking hormonal therapy drugs such as tamoxifen should talk to their doctors before trying to become pregnant, as these drugs could affect a developing fetus.

## Quality of Life

Women, who have undergone treatment for breast cancer should be reassured that their quality of life, once treatment has been completed, can be normal. Extensive studies have shown this. Women who have had chemotherapy may have a slight decrease in certain areas of function.

Some studies suggest that younger women, who represent about one fourth of breast cancer survivors, tend to have more problems adjusting to the stresses of breast cancer and its treatment. They have more psychosocial problems and trouble with emotional and social functioning. Some can feel isolated. Chemotherapy might have caused early menopause which requires adjustment. There may also be sexual difficulties. All these may need help with counseling and support groups directed to younger breast cancer survivors.

# Emotional Aspects of Breast Cancer[98]

It is important that your focus on tests and treatments does not prevent you from considering your emotional, psychological and spiritual health as well.

## Body image

A woman's choice of treatment will likely be influenced by her age, the image she has of herself and her body and her hopes and fears. For example, some women may select breast-conserving surgery with radiation therapy over a mastectomy for cosmetic and body image reasons. On the other hand, some women who choose mastectomy may want the affected area removed, regardless of the effect on their body image. They may be more concerned about the effects of radiation therapy than body image.

Other issues that women worry about include hair loss from chemotherapy and skin changes of the breast from radiation therapy. In addition to these body changes, women may also be dealing with concerns about the outcome of their treatment. These are all genuine concerns that affect how a woman makes decisions about her treatment, how she views herself, and how she feels about her treatment.

## Sexuality

Concerns about sexuality are often very worrisome to a woman with breast cancer. Several factors may place a woman at higher risk for sexual problems after breast cancer. It is important to remember that some treatments for breast cancer, such as chemotherapy, can change a woman's hormone levels and may negatively affect sexual interest and/or response. A diagnosis of breast cancer when a woman is in her twenties or thirties is especially difficult because choosing a partner and childbearing are often very important during this period.

Relationship issues are also important because the diagnosis can be very distressing for the partner, as well as the patient. Partners are usually concerned about how to express their love physically and emotionally after treatment, especially surgery.

Suggestions that may help a woman adjust to changes in her body image include looking at and touching herself; seeking the support of others, preferably before surgery; involving her partner as soon as possible after surgery; and openly communicating feelings, needs, and wants created by her changed image.

Sexual impact of surgery and radiation: Because breast cancer is the most common cancer in women (excluding skin cancer), sexual problems have been linked to mastectomy more often than to any other cancer treatment. Losing a breast, or occasionally both breasts if a woman later has a second tumor, can be traumatic.

The most common sexual side effects stem from damage to a woman's feelings of attractiveness. In our culture, we are taught to view breasts as a basic part of beauty and feminity. If her breast has been removed, a woman may be insecure about whether her partner will accept her and find her sexually pleasing.

The breasts and nipples are also sources of sexual pleasure for many women. Touching the breasts is a common part of foreplay in our culture. A few women can reach orgasm just from the stroking of their breasts. For many others, breast stimulation adds to sexual excitement.

Breast surgery or radiation to the breasts does not physically decrease a woman's sexual desire. Nor does it decrease her ability to have vaginal lubrication, normal genital feelings, or reach orgasm. Some good news from recent research is that within a year after their surgery, most women with early stage breast cancer have good emotional adjustment and sexual satisfaction. They report a quality of life similar to women who never had cancer.

Treatment for breast cancer can interfere with pleasure from breast caressing. After a mastectomy, the whole breast is gone. Some women still enjoy being stroked around the area of the healed scar. Others dislike being touched there and may no longer even enjoy being touched on the remaining breast and nipple.

Some women who have had a mastectomy feel self-conscious being the partner 'on top' during sex. The area of the missing breast is more visible in that position.

A few women have chronic pain in their chests and shoulders after radical mastectomy. During intercourse, supporting these areas with pillows may help. Also, avoid positions where your weight rests on your chest or arms.

If surgery removed only the tumor (segmental mastectomy or lumpectomy) and was followed by radiation therapy, the breast may still be scarred. It also may be a different shape or size. During radiation therapy, the skin may become red and swollen. The breast also may be a little tender. Breast and nipple feeling, however, should remain normal.

## Sexual impact of breast reconstruction

Breast reconstruction restores the shape of the breast, but it cannot restore normal breast sensation. The nerve that supplies feeling to the nipple runs through the deep breast tissue, and it gets disconnected during surgery. In a reconstructed breast, the feeling of pleasure from touching the nipple is lost. A rebuilt nipple has much less feeling.

In time, the skin on the reconstructed breast will regain some sensitivity but probably will not give the same kind of pleasure as before mastectomy. Breast reconstruction often makes women more comfortable with their bodies, however, and helps them feel more attractive.

## Effect on your partner

Breast cancer can be a growth experience for couples under certain circumstances. The relationship may be enhanced if the partner participates in decision making, and accompanies the woman to surgery and perhaps other treatments.

### About breast forms and bras

For women who have had a mastectomy, breast forms are an important alternative to breast reconstruction. Some women may not want further surgery, knowing that breast reconstruction can require several procedures to complete.

## Hormone Replacement Therapy after Breast Cancer

The known link between estrogen levels and breast cancer growth has discouraged many women and their doctors from choosing or recommending hormone replacement therapy (HRT). Unfortunately, many women experience menopausal symptoms after treatment for breast cancer. This can occur naturally or develop as a result of menopausal women stopping HRT. Chemotherapy can also cause early menopause in premenopausal women.

In the past, doctors have offered HRT after breast cancer treatment to women suffering from severe symptoms because early studies had shown no harm. However, in early 2004 a well-designed study (the HABITS study) found that breast cancer survivors taking HRT were much more likely to develop a new or recurrent breast cancer than women who were not taking the drugs. For this reason, most doctors now feel that for women previously treated for breast cancer, taking HRT would be unwise.

Women should consider discussing with their doctors alternatives to HRT pills to help with specific menopausal symptoms. Some doctors have suggested that phytoestrogens (estrogen-like substances from certain plant sources such as soy products) may be safer than the estrogens used in HRT. However, there is not enough information available on phytoestrogens to evaluate their safety for breast cancer survivors.

Chapter 15

# What is Counseling?

'Counseling' means different things to different people. The word is used to describe anything from a cup of tea and a chat with a friend, to seeing a psychotherapist three times a week.[101]

## What do we mean by counseling?

By counseling, we mean talking to someone who is properly trained. The person may be called a counselor or a psychotherapist. The difference between these two is sometimes difficult to distinguish. Some people use the terms to mean the same thing, as much of their work does overlap. The differences are usually to do with the type of training and special interests of the individual counselor or psychotherapist.

Whether you see a counselor or a psychotherapist doesn't usually matter. What matters is that they have done the appropriate training. Some other professionals (for example, GPs, nurses, psychologists, psychiatrists, social workers) may have been trained in counseling as well. But not all have, so it is important to check this out.

## Why do people have counseling?

There are many times in our lives when we all really feel we need someone to listen to us. This is basically what counseling is - someone listening to you. Being heard properly can be really important if you have cancer. You're probably finding it difficult to deal with the diagnosis. And you may be feeling a bit lost amongst all the treatments and doctors' appointments.

Most people feel very shocked when they are told they have cancer. It can turn your life 'upside down'. Things you can normally cope with, such as going to work, shopping, looking after the kids and socializing, may become more difficult, and have less meaning for you. Your intimate relationships might change because of changes in how you look and the way you feel about yourself. The stress you're under may mean you can't show the love and attention you want from your partner or children.

You may want to continue with life as normal, but feel frustrated that you can't. Many people with cancer have confusing and upsetting feelings such as anger and sadness and feelings that you're not in control of your life at this time can be very upsetting.

It's not uncommon to worry that your cancer could come back again after your treatment has finished or you may fear you are going to die. All of these feelings are very real and frightening. There's only so much your mind can process at one time, so these feelings can become overwhelming.

Bottling up feelings can become very draining and make living your life very difficult. Counseling gives you an opportunity to explore your feelings and express them in a safe place. A counselor can help you to find a way to make things less difficult to deal with.

If you're a relative of someone with cancer, you could probably do with spending a bit of time thinking about yourself in the midst of everything else. You are bound to have feelings of your own which you don't want to burden your sick loved one with. Being able to express your feelings may help you to support your relative more effectively.

Usually, you see a counselor for an hour at a regular time every week. You may have a weekly session for a set period of time (often six or eight weeks), or you might have sessions for as long as you and your counselor agree that you need them.

## Your counselor will try to

- Listen properly to what you are saying
- Not interrupt you

- Help you sort out and untangle your feelings and worries
- Provide you with insight into how you really think and feel
- Help you express your emotions in your own way
- Help you work out your own solutions to problems
- Help you accept what cannot be changed
- Help and support you while you do all this

Regular psychological counseling for breast cancer patients may do more than just lower their stress and anxiety. It can also mean healthier diets, reduced smoking, and most surprising of all—a stronger immune system.

## Tips for care givers [102]

The caregiver is typically a non-professional, trained family member, spouse or friend. Caregivers will be forced to learn new skills, take on new roles in the home and oftentimes provide financially for the family. Caregivers can easily become overwhelmed and experience sleep disorders, social withdrawal, feelings of guilt, anxiety, fatigue and depression. Several research studies have shown that the stress experienced by caregivers is lessened when they become educated about the disease, the treatment and how to meet the day-to-day needs of the cancer patient.

## Support systems

As you go through the process of coping with a diagnosis of breast cancer, you'll likely need different kinds of support from different people. For example, your healthcare team can support you medically. Your family or friends can offer emotional support. Religion may support you spiritually. Helpers can provide practical support with transportation or household tasks. You, yourself, may be a source of comfort or financial support for others, but you may find that you need help coping with these parts of life.

You'll also likely find that different concerns arise at the different stages of your healing. When you first learn you have breast cancer, you may have an almost overwhelming need for information. We intend that this Guide provide you with a foundation, helping you to access material that educates you about this illness. Once that need is satisfied, you may find that you have an important need to connect with other women who have recently gone through treatment. You may want to hear from a survivor about what it feels like to go through treatment. You may want to know whether your emotions are 'normal' or feel a need to voice your fears to someone who listens well.

You can connect with emotional and spiritual support through a variety of outlets.

You're already familiar with the support that family, friends, neighbors and co-workers can offer. Emotional and practical support can be wonderfully helpful and can bathe you in warmth and comfort. It can also be stressful.

People who don't have cancer can sometimes say foolish or hurtful things, or act in a way that doesn't feel at all helpful to you. You may feel angry, resentful, amused, happy and sad, all at the same time, while you watch them almost trip over themselves trying to offer you comfort. You'll feel better and so will they, if you can let people know exactly what you need, and whether and how you prefer to be helped.

Another avenue of support is a formal support group, which you can find at hospitals, health clinics and through online (internet) discussion groups, to name just a few. Several healthcare researchers have done scientific studies that show positive, sometimes life-extending benefits, for breast cancer patients who participate in support groups.

Support groups are not all alike. Some, such as self-help groups, tend to be loosely organized. While members meet at a set time on a regular schedule, the group is open to new members who might want to drop in to find out what the group is all about. The agenda of a meeting is fairly unstructured so that members can talk about whatever comes up. A professional may be involved in the administration of the group or in securing speakers, but the professional doesn't run the group. People (and most of them will be women in a breast cancer

# What is Counseling?

group) will likely be at different stages of recovery. Members will come and go as they feel the need. The group doesn't have a start and end date.

Information and coping skills groups are usually more structured. Group members begin and end sessions together and usually meet for a fixed period of time to deal with a specific concern. These groups are usually led by a professional: a psychologist, counselor, nurse, social worker, or doctor. A common format for such a group is to meet for two hours a week for eight or ten weeks. Some reasons for the group members to meet are to learn stress reduction skills, cope with uncertainty, learn about what foods to eat to be as healthy as possible, communicate, learn to take care of themselves and of each other or maintain emotional support. You don't usually drop in on these groups when you feel like it. Instead, you agree to go through a learning process with the same people for the same period of time.

Supportive therapy groups are long-term groups run by a mental health professional for a small number of women (usually six to eight) committed to the group. These groups focus on how to express emotions and provide mutual support.

In a buddy system, a woman who has been through breast cancer is paired up to offer one-on-one support to a woman who just found out she has breast cancer. Many hospitals have their own programs. How much support you receive from a buddy depends on what you want and need.

Formal group support doesn't work for everyone. Some women don't know what they would do without their group and others feel dissatisfied or disconnected from the groups.

If you find that groups don't work for you, you might consider looking into a buddy system or individual counseling.

Individual counseling is another way for you to obtain the emotional support you need while you cope with this diagnosis. Though many people believe that this sort of counseling is only for people with severe mental health problems, they are wrong.

For most people, a diagnosis of cancer is a trauma, something that hurts deeply and profoundly. It doesn't mean that there is something wrong with you that you need help to cope. In fact, it's a sign of health for you to recognize when you can't do something alone. It's okay to reach out.

Individual counselors come from a variety of backgrounds and follow a variety of approaches in the work they do. Some focus on behavior; others, on gaining insight into what makes you who you are; and still others, on providing emotional support while you heal. Many counselors combine approaches. Before you agree to work one-on-one, ask a counselor which approach she or he uses so that you can decide if that style fits your style.

Your health insurer, especially a managed care company, may limit the choices you have for covered individual counseling. Some contract with a particular mental health group or with a network of counselors in a specific geographic area. Your insurer may also limit the amount of payment available for counseling services. It's a good idea to check your health insurance plan for benefits before you make an appointment with a counselor.

Another source of counseling may be your religious advisor. Many women find that a diagnosis of cancer brings about a spiritual crisis. It's quite common to ask 'Why me?' Your spiritual counselor can offer you support in sorting through some of the deep concerns that can arise about your religion or values.

Many women are able to cope with the diagnosis and treatment of breast cancer with just the help of their close friends and family members. Others find they need a little more support, either in the form of support groups, individual counseling or financial assistance. Please keep in mind that it is always wise to know when to ask for help so that you can be as happy and healthy as possible.

It should be evident by now that you have many sources of support to consider. There is no one right way to deal with this situation. As with everything else in coping with breast cancer, don't let anyone tell you what you need or how you ought to feel or cope with this challenge. It's important for you to identify what you need, what you prefer, and what your limits are.

## Genetic counseling and breast cancer [103]

Not long ago, breast cancer was shrouded in mystery. Though doctors knew it affected the human body and had a number of fairly effective treatments, they knew little about its cause. The same could be said for the factors that affect risk. Now, however, thanks to recent advances in genetics, this is all changing, and quickly.

Today medical scientists can pinpoint mutations in individual genes which increase breast cancer risk. While these mutations do not account for all cases of breast cancer, there are other factors remaining to be explored. The presence of the mutations offers a more accurate picture of a person's risk for breast cancer. Some of these mutations are passed down through families and ethnic groups. For many women, this has important implications for monitoring, prevention and even treatment of breast and other cancers, such as ovarian cancer.

The risk from familial tendency can be expressed in this way: first degree relatives of breast cancer patients and fraternal twins have about 1.7 times the usual risk of developing breast cancer, while identical twins have about 4.4 times the usual risk.

The prevalence of inherited BRCA1 and BRCA2 mutations in the world population is lower, 0.1 to 0.2 percent. These mutations are implicated in about 10 percent of all cases of breast cancer. However, the numbers can change quite a lot, depending on an individual woman's history and circumstances. For instance, in women under forty who have breast cancer and who also have close relatives with breast cancer, approximately 75 percent carry these mutations.

## Genetic counseling [104,105,106,107,108,109,110,111]

Genetic testing is done to see if anyone of these mutations is present. Recent advances in genetics now enable to gain a much clearer picture about the risks of developing cancers such as breast and ovarian cancer. Armed with this knowledge, concerned individuals can consult their doctor and work out a program of close monitoring.

A more difficult issue is how to use the results in making decisions about monitoring, prevention or treatment. Before testing, a patient must be informed about and have a clear understanding of the risks and benefits of genetic testing. Genetic counseling should be offered before testing as well as after the results are received.

In addition, to breast cancer, mutations in BRCA2 may also confer as much as a 27 percent risk of ovarian cancer by age 70. And the increased risk does not stop, even after a woman has had an episode of cancer. These mutations also seem to significantly increase a woman's risk of developing a second case of breast cancer (or ovarian cancer) within five years of a first case, as compared to those of a woman without the mutation who has also had breast cancer. According to studies, the mutation carries up to a 6 percent risk of male breast cancer and an 8 percent risk of prostate cancer by age seventy, as well as increased (albeit low) risks for some other cancers. Men may also pass it on to their sons and daughters, who also may benefit from being screened. This is a particularly important point because in many families, breast cancer information is shared only among the women; many men may be unaware that they or their children are at risk.

The genes, known as BRCA1 and BRCA2, hold the key to genetic testing for breast cancer. Mutations of these genes account for about 80 percent of inherited breast cancers, and also signal an increased risk of ovarian cancer.

Genetic testing requires only a small blood sample from the patient. However, the test itself involves sophisticated molecular techniques in which DNA is extracted from white blood cells and is then sequenced. Only one laboratory in the nation conducts full DNA sequencing.

## Genetic counseling is crucial

Before DNA testing is performed, all patients undergo pre-test genetic counseling. Pre-test counseling involves assessment of the patient's personal and family medical history, education about basic genetics and cancer genetics and risk, and an in-depth discussion of the risks, benefits and limitations of testing. At the counseling sessions, misconceptions about breast and ovarian cancer risks are addressed. Sometimes patients believe they are at a much higher risk of cancer than they actually are.

Risk assessment is based on family history, including cousins, aunts, uncles and grandparents and medical records are obtained documenting cancer cases when possible. Risk factors for hereditary breast cancer include multiple cases of breast or ovarian cancer on one side of the family; cancer at an early age; cancer in both breasts, or breast and ovarian cancer, in the same individual; and male breast cancer. Patients of Ashkenazi Jewish ethnicity are at increased risk, as well. There are other risk factors for breast cancer such as bearing a first child after age thirty or never having had a child. But for someone with a family history suggestive of hereditary cancer, family history can overshadow such risk factors.

Ideally, genetic testing will begin with a family member who has cancer to identify if he or she carries a BRCA1 or BRCA2 mutation, which, therefore, is the likely cause of cancer in the family. If a healthy family member then tests negative for the mutated gene, her breast cancer risk is considered to be that of a woman in the general population: 12 percent lifetime risk of developing breast cancer and a 1-2 percent lifetime risk of developing ovarian cancer. If a healthy family member tests positive for the gene mutation identified in her family, she has a 60-80 percent lifetime risk of developing breast cancer and a 20-40 percent lifetime risk of developing ovarian cancer.

If a patient tests positive for a gene mutation, she will be followed more closely. Instead of an annual mammogram after the of age forty, she may begin annual mammograms ten years before the age of breast cancer onset in her relatives, in addition to a monthly self-examination and annual clinical breast examination. Annual ovarian cancer screening may be recommended, including a transvaginal ultrasound and CA125 blood test. Some women may choose to have their breasts and/or ovaries removed while still healthy as a preventive measure. Others may begin taking tamoxifen, a drug to prevent breast cancer.

## Impact of genetic testing

Genetic testing involves very personal decisions. Some patients feel empowered by knowing their genetic risk, while others prefer not to know or don't feel the additional information will be helpful.

Genetic counseling helps patients prepare for DNA test results and understand the psychological impact test results may have on their family and relationships. Some patients testing positive for a gene mutation may actually feel relief that the cause of breast cancer in their family has been identified and they have a diagnosis that can be dealt with. Some patients may require psychological counseling to address cancer fears. Others may be concerned about passing along the gene to their children. Some might be worried about insurance or job discrimination based on the diagnosis, although no such cases have yet been reported.

Testing negative for a gene mutation may provide relief, but it may even provide disappointment, as the cause of a family's breast cancers remains unknown. There may even be 'survivor guilt,' as one family member may feel guilty about not carrying a gene mutation while another does.

While genetic testing is not for everyone, the information provided in the counseling process is valuable for all patients.

## Patients report many barriers to counseling[112]

The researchers suggest that while more diligent doctors discuss psychosocial concerns with their patients and describe how counseling can help, others may just provide a brochure for the counseling center in a large packet of treatment-related information.

According to the study, the most commonly reported barriers to using counseling services were having adequate support (32%), lack of awareness of the service (25%) and lack of provider referral (13%). The results suggest that in addition to physician referral, education, social support, and spirituality may also influence the use of cancer support services.

## Patients need more education, referrals

The study also suggests the need for more systematic ways of educating patients about and providing referrals for counseling to cancer patients. In addition, the study showed that while oncologists think highly of cancer support services and report recommending them to a large percentage of their patients, few patients actually partake of the services. Cancer support services are generally not incorporated into oncology care in a systematic way; thus oncologists don't realize how few of their patients are using these services.

Chapter 16

# Recurrence of Breast Cancer

Breast cancer can recur at any time, but most recurrences occur in the first three to five years after initial treatment. Breast cancer can come back as a local recurrence (in the treated breast or near the mastectomy scar) or as a distant recurrence somewhere else in the body. The most common sites of recurrence include the lymph nodes, the bones, liver, or lungs.[113]

- ## What is secondary breast cancer?

A cancer is made up of millions of cancer cells. These form a tumor. Some cells may break away and spread to another part of the body and form a new tumor. Your doctor may call the new tumor a 'metastasis' or a 'secondary'. The original cancer is known as a 'primary' tumor or the 'primary' cancer.

So a secondary breast cancer is when the cancer which started in the breast has spread to another part of the body. The secondary cancer is made of the same type of cells as the primary cancer. So if a woman has secondary breast cancer in her bones, for example, she has breast cancer cells which have spread from her breast and formed another tumor in a bone.

This is different from having a cancer that first started in the bone (a primary bone cancer). In that case, the cancer is made up of bone cells that have become cancerous.

Secondary breast cancer can appear differently in different women. For example, a woman with secondary breast cancer affecting a bone will have different symptoms from a woman with secondary breast cancer affecting her liver. This is because, although their bones and liver are affected by the same type of cancer cells, their growth will have different effects in different parts of the body.

## How breast cancer cells spread

If cancer cells spread from primary breast cancer, there are two ways they can travel to another part of the body:

- In the bloodstream
- In the lymph fluid which flows through the lymphatic system

Once they move around the body, the cancer cells can be trapped in different organs and tissues. Then they may grow and divide to form a secondary breast cancer. But breast cancer cells do not always form a secondary cancer as soon as they have found a new site. Often they die. Sometimes they are inactive for many years. No one knows why some cancer cells stay inactive or what can start them years later to form a secondary cancer.

## Types of recurrences [114]

Occasionally breast cancer can return after primary treatment. There are three types of recurrent breast cancer:

- Local recurrence: Cancerous tumor cells remain in the original site, and over time, grow back. Most physicians do not consider local breast cancer recurrence to be the spread of breast cancer, but rather, failure of the primary treatment. Even after mastectomy (surgical removal of the affected breast), portions of the breast skin and fat remain, and local recurrence is possible (however, it is uncommon).
- Regional recurrence: A regional recurrence of breast cancer is more serious than local recurrence because it usually indicates that the cancer has spread past the breast and the axillary (underarm) lymph nodes. Regional breast cancer recurrences can

occur in the pectoral (chest) muscles, in the internal mammary lymph nodes under the breastbone and between the ribs, in the supraclavicular nodes (above the collarbone), and in the nodes surrounding the neck.

- Distant recurrence: A distant breast cancer recurrence, also known as a metastasis (spread), is the most dangerous type of recurrence. Once out of the breast, cancer usually spreads first to the axillary (underarm) lymph nodes. In 25 percent of distant recurrences, breast cancer spreads from the lymph nodes to bone. Other sites breast cancer may spread to include the bone marrow, lungs, liver, brain, or other organs.

Often, a diagnosis of recurrent cancer is more devastating or psychologically difficult for a woman than her initial breast cancer diagnosis. Women who have recurrent breast cancer are encouraged to discuss their feelings with a counselor or therapist and consider joining a support group.

## Local and regional recurrence

Breast cancer most commonly recurs in the same area as the original cancer had occurred. Women with ductal carcinoma in situ (DCIS) who are treated with breast-conserving therapy (lumpectomy and radiation) are at a slightly higher risk of experiencing a recurrence than those women who are treated with mastectomy (removal of the affected breast). However, several studies have shown that women treated with breast conserving therapy who have local recurrence of DCIS are not at any significantly greater risk of dying from the disease than women treated with mastectomy. DCIS is a common type of cancer that is confined to the milk ducts of the breast.

A recurrence of non-invasive breast cancer is less serious than a recurrence of invasive cancer. In general, invasive local recurrences are more aggressive since they have a second chance of spreading (metastasizing) to other areas of the body.

Once recurrent breast cancer has been detected, physicians will order additional tests to determine to what extent the cancer has spread. These tests may include: bone scan, chest X-ray, CAT scan,

MRI scan, and liver blood tests. Treatment of a local recurrence often depends on how the initial treatment was performed. If lumpectomy was performed, recurrent breast cancer will usually be treated with mastectomy.

A local recurrence after mastectomy will usually present itself as a small lump in the mastectomy scar or under the skin. This type of recurrence often goes undetected for some time because it may be mistaken for a leftover stitch or scar tissue from the mastectomy operation. Once the lump grows, breast biopsy is performed to determine whether it is cancerous.

Breast reconstruction rarely hides recurrent breast cancer. Local recurrences with implants are most often in front of the implant, and recurrences with TRAM flap procedures are along the edge of the breast skin (not in the flap).

Women whose initial breast cancer was aggressive are more likely to have recurrences than other women. Inflammatory breast cancer with cancer cells in the lymphatics of the skin or breast often recurs. (Lymphatics are key components of the body's immune system). Also, women with large tumors or several cancerous lymph nodes may experience recurrent breast cancer. Often, these types of recurrent cancers are treated with mastectomy (if it was not performed during primary treatment) followed by radiation therapy to the chest wall.

Regional breast cancer recurrences are rare, occurring in approximately 2 percent of all breast cancer cases. Most often, regional recurrence appears as a cancerous axillary (underarm) lymph node that was not removed during primary treatment. Treatment involves simply removing the cancerous node. Regional recurrence in the lymph nodes of the neck or above the collarbone usually indicates more aggressive cancers.

Besides local and regional recurrences, a new cancer may occasionally occur years after the initial cancer. Usually, the new cancer is in a different area of the breast and does not have the same pathology. For example, the original cancer is ductal carcinoma in situ (DCIS) and the second cancer appears invasive lobular carcinoma. Second cancers are treated as new cancers, independent of the first cancer.

## Distant recurrence

A distant recurrence of breast cancer is called metastatic disease. Metastatic breast cancer (Stage IV) is serious and the survival rate is considerably lower than for women whose cancer is confined to the breast or axillary (underarm) lymph nodes. Breast cancer has the potential to spread to almost any region of the body. The most common region is bone, followed by the lung and liver.

Symptoms of metastatic breast cancer may include:

- Bone pain (possible indication of bone metastases)
- Shortness of breath (possible indication of lung metastases)
- Lack of appetite (possible indication of liver metastases)
- Weight loss (possible indication of liver metastases)
- Neurological pain or weakness, headaches (possible indication of neurological metastases)

These symptoms are sometimes but not always associated with metastatic breast cancer. Additionally, having one or more of these symptoms does not necessarily mean a woman has metastatic breast cancer. Any changes in health should be reported to a physician for further examination. Metastatic breast cancer is usually diagnosed by bone scan, CAT scan, MRI scan, or liver blood tests.

Surgery is rarely an option for metastatic breast cancer because the cancer is not usually confined to one specific spot on the given organ. Instead, treatment options include one or more of the following: chemotherapy, radiation therapy, or hormonal (drug) therapies. Patients with advanced breast cancer may wish to consider entering into a clinical trial designed to evaluate the effectiveness of newly developed treatments.

## How do I know there is a recurrence?

If you've been treated for breast cancer, you should continue to practice breast self-examination, checking both the treated area and your other breast each month. You should report any changes to your doctor right away. Breast changes that might indicate a recurrence include:

- An area that is distinctly different from any other area on either breast
- Lump or thickening in or near the breast or in the underarm that persists through the menstrual cycle
- A change in the size, shape, or contour of the breast
- A mass or lump, which may feel as small as a pea
- A marble-like area under the skin
- A change in the feel or appearance of the skin on the breast or nipple, including skin that is dimpled, puckered, scaly, or inflamed (red, warm or swollen)
- Bloody or clear fluid discharge from the nipples
- Redness of the skin on the breast or nipple

In addition to performing monthly breast self-exams, keep your scheduled follow-up appointments with your healthcare provider. During these appointments, your healthcare provider will perform a breast exam, order lab or imaging tests as needed, and ask you about any symptoms you might have. Initially, these follow-up appointments may be scheduled every three to four months. The longer you are cancer-free, the less often you will need to see your healthcare provider. Continue to follow your healthcare provider's recommendations on screening mammograms (usually recommended once a year).

## What factors determine the likelihood of a recurrence?[113]

Prognostic indicators are characteristics of a patient and her tumor that may help a physician predict a cancer recurrence. These are some common indicators:

- **Lymph node involvement:** Women who have lymph node involvement are more likely to have a recurrence.
- **Tumor size:** In general, the larger the tumor, the greater the chance of recurrence.
- **Hormone receptors:** About two-thirds of all breast cancers contain significant levels of estrogen receptors, which means the

tumors are estrogen receptor positive (ER+). ER-positive tumors tend to grow less aggressively and may respond favorably to treatment with hormones.

- **Histologic grade:** This term refers to how much the tumor cells resemble normal cells when viewed under the microscope. The higher the histologic grade, the greater chance of recurrence.
- **Nuclear grade:** This is the rate at which cancer cells in the tumor divide to form more cells. Cancer cells with a high nuclear grade (also called proliferative capacity) are usually more aggressive (faster growing).
- **Oncogene expression:** An oncogene is a gene that causes or promotes cancerous changes within the cell. Tumors that contain certain oncogenes may increase a patient's chance of recurrence.

## How will my prognosis affect my treatment?

Following surgery or radiation, your treatment team will determine the likelihood that the cancer will recur outside the breast. This team usually includes a medical oncologist, a specialist trained in using medicines to treat breast cancer. The medical oncologist, who works with your surgeon, may advise the use of tamoxifen (tamoxifen citrate) or possibly chemotherapy. These treatments are used in addition to, but not in place of, local breast cancer treatment with surgery and/or radiation therapy.

## How would a recurrence be treated?[113]

The type of treatment for local breast cancer recurrences depends on your initial treatment. If you had a lumpectomy, local recurrence is usually treated with mastectomy. If the initial treatment was mastectomy, recurrence near the mastectomy site is treated by removing the tumor whenever possible, usually followed by radiation therapy.

In either case, hormone therapy and/or chemotherapy may be used after surgery and/or radiation therapy. If breast cancer is found in the other breast, it may be a new tumor unrelated to the first breast cancer. Treatment would include a lumpectomy or mastectomy and possibly radiation and/or systemic therapy (chemotherapy and/or hormonal therapy).

Women with distant recurrence involving organs such as the bones, lungs, brain or other organs are treated with systemic therapy. Radiation therapy or surgery may also be recommended to relieve certain symptoms.

Immunotherapy with trastuzumab (Herceptin) alone or with chemotherapy may be recommended for women whose cancer cells have high levels of the HER2/neu protein. Immunotherapy is generally started after hormonal or chemotherapy are no longer effective.

Chapter 17

# Breast Cancer in Men

In men, breast cancer is a rare disease. Men account for about 1 percent of breast cancers reported in the United States that is for every 100 cases of breast cancer, 99 are seen in females and only 1 in males,-- or 1,600 new cases last year, statistics in the US reveal. The breast cancer constitutes only 0.2 per cent of all malignancies seen in males whereas breast cancer is the commonest cancer in females–about 26 per cent. The American Cancer Society estimates that in 2003 some 1,300 new cases of invasive breast cancer was diagnosed among men in the US.

Breast cancer is about 100 times more common among women.

Estimates for 2003 also indicate that there were more than 40,000 deaths from breast cancer in the US (39,800 women, 400 men).

The average age at diagnosis is between 60 and 70, although men of all ages can be affected with the disease.

The median incidence in over 100 cancer registries world-wide is 0.5/1,00,000/year. However, several large case series have been reported in regions in Africa where breast cancer accounts for 6±15% of all male carcinomas.[115]

There are about 300 cases diagnosed each year in the UK, compared with almost 42,000 cases of breast cancer in women.[116] That's about one man for every 140 women diagnosed. Federal reports show the male death rate has remained steady at 0.3 per 1,00,000 men. In India, the incidence is still lower. Because of its rarity, clinicians and researchers have not been able to collect substantial data on the subject and ignorance persists both in the minds of the doctors and the public.[117]

Men who have breast cancer usually discover the disease later than women, when the tumors are larger and the cancer has spread, according to findings from the largest-ever study of male breast cancer.

Men with cancer were found to be older, more likely to have later-stage cancers that had spread to the lymph nodes, and more likely to have ductal and papillary cancers, the study says.

A majority of people are unaware that breast cancer can afflict men too.

The breast tissue is the same in males and females, and till puberty, boys and girls have a small amount of breast tissue (mainly ducts) under the nipple. At puberty, the hormonal status is vastly changed. An increase in female hormones gives rise to development of secondary sexual characters, the breasts start enlarging in size, whereas in males the male hormones give rise to development of male secondary characters, the breasts hardly increase in size and thus the differentiation takes place.

Males also have a small quantity of estrogen, the main female sex hormone. The small quantity normally does not give rise to enlargement of breast tissue. Over production of estrogen, as seen in some diseases ( liver cirrhosis, cancer of the testes or adrenal glands, Klinefelter's syndrome (a syndrome in which males have an extra X chromosome) chronic renal failure of patients on dialysis, can give rise to enlargement of breasts in the same fashion as seen in females and this enlargement is known as gynecomastia.

This is also known to occur after the use of certain medicines. The well-documented ones are the drugs used for ulcers, blood pressure, heart failure, migraine, seizures, and also the use of estrogen commonly prescribed for cancer of prostate. Forty per cent of adolescent boys do experience gynecomastia but it soon disappears. During old age, when the hormonal balance changes, the breast size may enlarge. The accumulation of fat in obese men (a classical example is Sumo wrestlers) can make the breasts appear enlarged but this is not true gynecomastia.

The male breast cancer patients are diagnosed at an advanced stage of the disease, even in developed countries; this delay results in bad prognosis of the male breast cancer patients as compared to females. The small size of the male breast also contributes.

Breast tumor tissue contains hormone receptors in a high proportion of men–over 80 percent as compared to 65 percent in women but because of the paucity of vast experience on the subject, it is not yet known if positive hormone receptor status indicates a better prognosis as seen in women. Similarly the role of antiestrogen agents has not been well established although it is considered to be beneficial. Surgical castration has been also credited to give beneficial results – regression of the size of the tumor, relief of symptoms and clearance of metastasis in a few patients but the experience is scanty. A patient of male breast cancer may go into a state of depression particularly if he considers himself to be harboring a disease that is predominantly for females, and one that involves hormone imbalances; this might be perceived as a threat to his masculinity. He definitely requires support and sympathy from his dear and near ones. [118,119,120]

## Risks and causes[121]

As with women, the single biggest risk factor for male breast cancer is increasing age. Most cases are diagnosed in men between the ages of 60 and 70. Other risk factors are:

- High estrogen levels
- Exposure to radiation
- Family history or recognized breast cancer gene in the family
- A rare genetic condition called Klinefelter's syndrome

All men produce some estrogen. This is perfectly normal. But high estrogen levels have been linked to breast cancer. High estrogen levels can occur in:

- Obesity–estrogen is partly made in the fat (adipose) tissues of the body
- Chronic liver conditions, such as cirrhosis
- Genetic conditions

Men, who have been exposed to radiation repeatedly, over a long period of time, are more likely to develop male breast cancer. This is particularly true if they were young when the radiation exposure took place.

There is an increased risk of breast cancer in men with women in their family who have already been diagnosed with breast cancer. This is particularly true if the women are close relations (mother or sisters). And if the women were diagnosed at a young age (below forty). Men, as well as women, can inherit faulty genes that can cause breast cancer. Between five and ten out of every hundred (5 – 10%) breast cancers diagnosed in women are thought to be due directly to an inherited faulty gene. In men, this may be more common. We think that between ten and twenty out of every hundred diagnosed (10 – 20%) are due to inherited faulty genes.

Klinefelter's syndrome is a rare genetic condition where a man is born with an extra female chromosome. So he is XXY instead of XY. Men with Klinefelter's are about 20 times more likely to get breast cancer than the average man. This makes their breast cancer risk the same as for the average woman.

## Symptoms

The commonest symptom for men with breast cancer is a lump in the breast area. This is nearly always painless. Other symptoms can include:

- Oozing from the nipple (a discharge) that may be blood stained
- Swelling of the breast
- A sore (ulcer) in the skin of the breast
- A nipple that is pulled into the breast (called nipple retraction)
- Lumps under the arm

Male breast cancer is a disease in which malignant (cancer) cells form in the tissues of the breast. Men at any age may develop breast cancer, but it is usually detected (found) in men between sixty and seventy years of age.

## Types of breast cancer found in men:[122]

- **Infiltrating ductal carcinoma:** Cancer that has spread beyond the cells lining ducts in the breast. Most men with breast cancer have this type of cancer.
- **Ductal carcinoma in situ:** Abnormal cells that are found in the lining of a duct; also called intraductal carcinoma.
- **Inflammatory breast cancer:** A type of cancer in which the breast looks red and swollen and feels warm.
- **Paget's disease of the nipple:** A tumor that has grown from ducts beneath the nipple onto the surface of the nipple.

Lobular carcinoma in situ (abnormal cells found in one of the lobes or sections of the breast), which sometimes occurs in women, has not been seen in men.

## What are the similarities with breast cancer in women?

Lymph node involvement and the hematogenous pattern of spread are similar to those found in female breast cancer. The staging system for male breast cancer is identical to the staging system for female breast cancer.

Prognostic factors that have been evaluated include the size of lesion and the presence or absence of lymph node involvement, both of which correlate well with prognosis.

- Overall survival is similar to that of women with breast cancer. The impression that male breast cancer has a worse prognosis may stem from the tendency towards diagnosis at a later stage.

Some men with breast cancer feel that the information available is biased towards women. That is understandable, but when you look at the figures, you can see why breast cancer information is aimed at women.

The important thing is that most of the information men with breast cancer need is the same. The symptoms, diagnosis and treatment are all very similar to women with breast cancer. Obviously there are areas where women need different information than men on reconstruction or the different types of breast shapes (prostheses) available.

The tests used to diagnose breast cancer in men are much the same as for women. The same treatments are used for breast cancer in men as for women.

## Finding support

Of course it is difficult for anyone diagnosed with breast cancer. But it can be particularly difficult for men, as they may feel very confused and isolated. It is so common to hear about breast cancer in women. But not at all common to hear about it in men. So it can be difficult even to believe that the diagnosis is right. As male breast cancer is rare, men are often treated in large, specialist centres where there is expertise in dealing with the disease.

Survival for men with breast cancer is similar to that for women with breast cancer when their stage at diagnosis is the same. Breast cancer in men, however, is often diagnosed at a later stage. Cancer found at a later stage may be less likely to be cured.

Certain factors affect prognosis (chance of recovery) and treatment options.

## Prognosis

It depends on the following:
- The stage of the cancer (whether it is in the breast only or has spread to other places in the body)
- The type of breast cancer
- Certain characteristics of the cancer cells
- Whether the cancer is found in the other breast
- The patient's age and general health

## Recurrent male breast cancer

Recurrent breast cancer is cancer that has recurred (come back) after it has been treated. The cancer may come back in the breast, in the chest wall, or in other parts of the body.

Any initiative should include:

1. The development and implementation of a structured education program aimed primarily at all health-care professionals and a well-publicized media initiative to raise awareness about male breast cancer and its treatment.
2. The availability of gender-specific information both pre and postoperatively to help to alleviate the potential psychological problems associated with the diagnosis of cancer.
3. The provision of appropriate counseling services for the wives of male patients and possibly encouragement of breast care nurses to establish supportive relationships with those affected men who might consider a 'female support' less threatening than a male.

Chapter 18

# Alternative Therapies for Breast Cancer Treatment

## Complementary and Alternative Medicine (CAM)

Complementary and alternative medicine(CAM) includes a wide array of healing philosophies, therapies, and approaches. Complementary and alternative medicine is a group of diverse medical and health care systems, practices, and products that are not presently considered to be part of conventional medicine.[123,124,125] While some scientific evidence exists regarding some CAM therapies, for most there are key questions that are yet to be answered through well-designed scientific studies–questions such as whether these therapies are safe and whether they work for the diseases or medical conditions for which they are used.

Complementary therapies are those used in addition to conventional treatment, whereas alternative treatments are used instead of standard care. Depending on utilization techniques, some approaches may be considered either complementary or alternative. Research focusing on CAM use by women with breast cancer is a relatively new field of study. The scientific efficacy of most CAM interventions is unknown. A patient's perceptions and understanding of his/her illness is an evolving process that may have an influence on quality of life and health behavior choices.[126] Distress levels seem higher among women who choose CAM as part of their health surveillance regimen, perhaps indicating that this group is seeking additional coping mechanisms. It has also been suggested that the true appeal in CAM may be the sense of hope and self-control felt by the patient who chooses CAM modalities.[127] It remains to be discovered whether this feeling of empowerment actually provides any true medical benefit.[128]

Decisions to use CAM are highly individualized, complicated. The decision to use–or not to use–CAM is not a one-time decision; instead, it is a decision that leads cancer patients to reflect on their unique personal and social context and to ponder how CAM may fit with their values, beliefs, and specific health care needs.

Despite the need for additional research and professional education on CAM, it is essential that oncology health professionals begin a dialogue with patients that focuses not just on individual CAM therapies, but also on how to make treatment decisions that acknowledge scientific evidence and each patient's beliefs, values, and sociocultural contexts.[129]

# Yoga

Yoga, the ancient Indian therapy for exercise and meditation of the mind and the body, has for long been known to help people cope against ailments. And now, the age old therapy is providing a healing touch to patients suffering from breast cancer by reducing pain and trauma.

The University of Texas MD Anderson Cancer Centre and the Swami Vivekananda Yoga Anusandhana Samsthana, have announced a research collaboration to scientifically validate the belief that mind-body interventions have a beneficial impact on the health of cancer patients. The University of Texas, MD Anderson Cancer Centre is the world's largest cancer hospital and research centre. Dr H R Nagendra, the President of 'Swami Vivekananda Yoga Anusandhana Samsthana' has said that the research on breast cancer patients through specially developed Yoga technique helped control their agony, adding that the MD Anderson Centre has accepted the theory.

'Yoga is an effective agent and it can bring a lot of improvement for the patients. For the last twenty-five years we have been doing extensive research, findings of which are published in nearly seventy-five research papers in the top journals. What we have been able to show is that yoga is effective by systematic protocols, which are acceptable by international standards. The MD Anderson Centre has also come forward and for the first time seen how yoga can be useful for cancer patients. They are very much impressed,' said Dr HR Nagendra. The ten-year research at Bangalore Institute of Oncology on Yoga therapy on more than 400 breast cancer patients has given a positive output and it is based on this research, that the MD Anderson Centre has accepted Yoga as a therapy for relieving pain in breast cancer patients.

Researchers from both institutions are currently studying the effects of yoga on breast cancer patients undergoing radiation treatments. They are also exploring whether participating in a yoga programme diminishes patients' fatigue and sleep disturbances, while improving the overall quality of life, mental health, stress hormone levels and aspects of immune function.

Specifically tailored yoga programs may help women with late-stage breast cancer by reducing pain and fatigue and raising their spirits, according to a pilot study published in the Journal of Pain and Symptom Management.[130]

In the study, Moadel and her colleagues studied 126 women undergoing chemotherapy for breast cancer. The average age of the women was fifty three and most of them had stage I or II breast cancer. Some were assigned to yoga classes and the rest to a yoga wait list comparison group.

The yoga program consisted of twelve weeks of classes three times a week and daily home practice sessions guided by audio tapes.

Overall, the women assigned to the yoga program had a 12 percent improvement in quality of life measurements, compared with women in the comparison group, says Moadel. In addition to improved sense of well-being, the women had less fatigue and better physical functioning, she says.

At the same time, the women in the comparison group said they were experiencing more social and emotional distress.[131]

In a new study of breast cancer survivors practicing Iyengar yoga–a form of yoga that incorporates all of the components of physical fitness and focuses on structural body alignment as well as mental relaxation has found that breast cancer survivors who practice yoga experience changes in the way their immune cells respond to activation signals. This may be important for understanding how physical activity and meditative practices benefit the immune system. The function of genes in immune cells can be regulated by proteins called transcription factors.

Restorative Yoga involves the combination of physical postures, breathing and deep relaxation. It has been described as 'active relaxation.' Patients with cancer often do not have the physical strength or mental energy for vigoros physical activity or more traditional types of yoga. Restorative poses can be very useful for people who feel weak, fatigued or highly stressed. Restorative Yoga is gentle enough that it can be practiced when a person is ill or recovering from surgery. By using props like bolsters, blankets, and straps (all provided) Students can ease themselves into postures that gently stretch the body and allow it to relax. Restorative Yoga moves the spine through its complete range of motion – forward, backward, sideways and twisted. It does but gently and is supported by props and assisted by the teacher. Deep relaxation in each of the postures is an important part of Restorative Yoga practice. As students rest in each gentle posture, they practice consciously releasing each muscle group and gently direct their thoughts to soothing ideas and images.[132]

Yoga is also associated with decreased post chemotherapy nausea and vomiting, decrease in post-chemotherapy nausea frequency and intensity and in the intensity of anticipatory nausea and vomiting.[133]

## Homeopathy

Homeopathy is based on the idea that if large doses of a substance cause a symptom, very small doses of that same substance will cure it. Homeopathic remedies are water (and sometimes alcohol) based solutions containing tiny amounts of certain naturally occurring plants, minerals, animal products or chemicals. The term 'homeopathy' comes from the Greek words 'homoios' (similar) and 'pathos' (suffering).

While homeopathy appears to be safe, there is little if any reliable clinical evidence that homeopathic remedies are effective in treating cancer or that they can help with the side effects of cancer or its treatment.

Homeopathy is most often promoted for use in treating chronic or self-limiting problems such as arthritis, asthma, colds, flu, and allergies. However, some supporters believe that homeopathy can be used to treat and cure cancer.

Some practitioners claim homeopathy can help cancer patients by reducing pain, improving vitality and well being, stopping the spread of cancer, and strengthening the immune system. Some claim it can lessen certain symptoms and side effects from radiation, chemotherapy, and hormone therapy, such as infections, nausea, vomiting, mouth sores, hot flushes, hair loss, depression, weakness, and ascites (collection of fluid in the abdomen).

Proponents claim that homeopathic solutions, even though they may contain very small quantities (or none) of the original ingredient, contain a 'memory' of the substance that somehow interacts with the body to cure illness. It is also believed that shaking or diluting a homeopathic solution releases the essence, or healing life force of the material.

Homeopathy is most often promoted for use in treating chronic or self-limiting problems such as arthritis, asthma, colds, flu, and allergies. However, some supporters believe that homeopathy can be used to treat and cure cancer.

Some practitioners claim homeopathy can help cancer patients by reducing pain, improving vitality and well being, stopping the spread of cancer, and strengthening the immune system. Some claim it can lessen certain symptoms and side effects of radiation, chemotherapy and hormone therapy, such as infections, nausea, vomiting, mouth sores, hot flushes, hair loss, depression, weakness, and ascites (collection of fluid in the abdomen).

## Chinese Medicine and Herbal Medicine

Traditional Chinese Medicine (TCM) is a comprehensive system of medical thought, pathophysiological concepts, and therapeutic interventions that developed in a period of Chinese civilization, spanning more than four thousand years. The primary modality of TCM is the use of an extensive pharmacopoeia of over 6,000 herbal and other natural products for the prevention and treatment of disease and the promotion of health.

TCM has four main components: acupuncture, herbal medicine, tui na, and qi gong. Herbal medicines are generally delivered in compound formulas specially formulated for a clinical syndrome or constellation of symptoms. Tui na is the ancient Chinese massage used for lymphatic drainage and muscle rejuvenation. Qi gong is the practice of energy movement in the body through physical movement. Herbal remedies have been around for thousands of years. Now, women with breast cancer facing chemotherapy and radiation are supplementing this traditional medicine with herbal remedies and alternative treatments. They are not abandoning the usual breast cancer treatment; they are using herbal remedies and alternative treatments to curb the side effects.[134]

Ginseng has been used by the Chinese for centuries. They believe that it stimulates the immune system and energizes the patient. There are more than thirty active compounds in the ginseng root. Many of the compounds are believed to have anti-tumor properties. In a Chinese study it was found that women who took ginseng before their diagnosis had a higher survival rate than the women who took ginseng after their diagnosis. Women have reported that they have a higher quality of life and suffer less depression while using ginseng.

There is a mushroom, the Maitake that helps in boosting the immune system. Here again, in the East this has been used widely. Lab studies have been done using liquid Maitake extract. Many researchers believe that the mushrooms contain beta-glucans which helps to enhance the immune system. They still don't know why, but they are working on it.

Mistletoe extract has been used in Europe to treat cancer patients for over eighty years. It has been shown to kill cancer cells and boost the immune system. There have been very few studies done here on mistletoe, but some research is under way and will be out at the end of this year. Researchers are studying the safety, the effects on the immune system and its toxicity. Mary Hanna is an aspiring herbalist who lives in Central Florida. Mary has also published articles on Cruising, Gardening and Cooking for more information on these subjects. Herbal agents are increasingly being investigated to address the debilitating side effects from conventional cancer treatment. Ginger (*Zingiber officinale*) may be effective in treating chemotherapy-induced nausea and vomiting (Manusirivithaya et al. 2004. Ginkgo (*Ginkgo biloba*), has been used to reduce the toxic side effects of some chemotherapeutic drugs. Evidence from in vivo studies show protective effects against nephrotoxicity induced by cisplatin and cardiotoxicity induced by doxorubicin. While clinical trials are not yet available to determine its effectiveness in practice, this aspect of herbal medicine in cancer patients represents large and diverse opportunities for positive integration into oncology patient management.

Astragalus (*Astragalus membranaceus*) has been used in cancer therapy to not only reduce the associated side effects but also to enhance the effectiveness of chemotherapy (Block and Mead 2003). A Cochrane systematic review of Chinese herbs for chemotherapy induced side-effects in colorectal patients analyzed the results of four trials that used a formulation containing astragalus (huang-qi). Despite study limitations, it was concluded that formulations of astragalus may stimulate immuno-competent cells and decrease side effects in patients treated with chemotherapy

One of the more problematic side effects of radiation therapy is the incidental damage to normal tissues. Damage to normal tissues, in some cases, can be sufficiently severe to stop radiation treatment. For example, acute radiation skin toxicity can cause such debilitating skin breakdown that the full course of radiation therapy cannot be completed. Wheatgrass extract has been shown to decrease the time to onset of the most severe grading of acute radiation skin toxicity, improving treatment compliance. There are other potential side effects, short and long term, that result from cancer treatment that might benefit from herbal medicine. While there is a lack of empirical evidence for support, the following might find a place in cancer management: analgesics (pain/palliation), antidepressant (compliance/recovery), antidiarrheal (abdominal radiotherapy), antiecchymotic (chemotherapy), antiemetric (chemotherapy, gut radiotherapy), antifibrotic (radiation damage), anti edematous (surgical or radiation damage), antioxidant (free radicals from radiotherapy), cathartic (constipation), collagen stabilising (radiation damage) and hypnotics (rest).[135]

## Acupuncture

Acupuncture is a component of the health care system of China that can be traced back for at least 2,500 years. The general theory of acupuncture is based on the premise that there are patterns of energy flow (qi) through the body that are essential for health. Disruptions of this flow are believed to be responsible for disease. Acupuncture is used to correct imbalances of qi flow at identifiable anatomical locations on and just below the skin, the acupuncture points, by the stimulation of a variety of techniques. The most studied mechanism of stimulation of acupuncture points employs penetration of the skin by thin, solid, specially tipped, metallic needles, which are manipulated manually or by electrical current.

Acupuncture is especially helpful for nausea and post surgical pain. Many studies done by research oncologists have shown that acupuncture was better for women with breast cancer than the medication taken to fight nausea. It also helps in loss of appetite, fatigue and sleep disorders. The AAMA recommends women with breast cancer should get acupuncture during their chemotherapy treatments but only after you have spoken to your primary doctor.[136]

All doctors and researchers stress that diet and exercise play a key role in treating cancer. Stick to a diet that is high in fruits, vegetables and grains. The National Cancer Institute recommends at least five servings of fresh fruits and vegetables per day. Phytochemicals are found in fruits and vegetables and they prevent cancers in a number of ways. Research shows that they help in detoxification of carcinogens, DNA repair, boosting of the immune system and maintenance of cellular control mechanisms. Obesity plays a role in getting cancer. Change your diet, eat healthy and go for a walk or ride a bike. This is a suggestion we should all take to heart.[137]

These alternative methods may well help you through your breast cancer treatment and perhaps even get you a speedier recovery. New studies are being done everyday for women with breast cancer. Discuss these alternative therapies with your doctor and always let your physician and your oncologist know about any therapies you want to take, before you take them. This will make sure that the alternative therapy won't interfere with your chemotherapy and radiation therapy.

## Meditation and Chanting

Meditation is a mental discipline by which one attempts to get beyond the reflexive, 'thinking' mind into a deeper state of relaxation or awareness. Meditation often involves turning attention to a single point of reference. It is recognized as a component of almost all religions, and has been practiced for over 5,000 years.[138,139] Meditation has been defined as: 'self regulation of attention, in the service of self-inquiry, in the here and now.'[140] In 1976, the Australian psychiatrist Ainslie Meares, reported in the Medical Journal of Australia, the regression of cancer following intensive meditation. People have used meditation to help treat a number of problems, including:[141]

- Anxiety, stress, and depression
- Pain
- Addictive behaviors such as using drugs, nicotine and alcohol; meditation may help with these problems, but it doesn't take the place of treatment you receive from a doctor

One of the great things about meditation is that you can do it on your own whenever you want, and it may help you relax and feel better. Also, you don't need any special tools or equipment to practice meditation.

Learning how to be aware of the present moment in meditation may keep your mind sharp and help you focus better in other areas of life as well. For example, you may be able to react faster to road conditions when you drive if you focus solely on driving, rather than being distracted by talking, thinking about other things, or listening to the radio.[142]

Chanting of Om reduces stress and has been tried for diabetes and hypertension.[143]

## Reiki

Reiki means 'universal life energy' and is an ancient healing method that manipulates energy flow in the body. Reiki practitioners believe there is an energy force in and around the body. They believe that there is a flow of energy between the reiki practitioner and the receiver of the treatment. It is thought that reiki releases energy flows and allows the body's own natural healing ability to work.

Reiki focuses on seven main energy centers, called chakras, in your body. The energy should flow freely through your chakras in order for you to be spiritually, physically and mentally healthy. Practitioners believe that if energy paths are blocked, you may feel ill or weak or have pain.

A reiki treatment session usually lasts an hour. The reiki practitioner puts his or her hands over or on your body at certain chakras. Most reiki practitioners recommend more than one session.

People use reiki to decrease pain, ease muscle tension, speed healing, and improve sleep.

Reiki is sometimes used to help people who suffer from pain or discomfort from cancer or other diseases. But reiki is not used as a treatment for cancer or any other disease. Some people who have undergone chemotherapy treatment said they felt better and had less nausea after undergoing a reiki session. Research is ongoing to determine any benefits of reiki.

Many people who receive reiki say they experience a refreshed spirit, better healing and an increase in general well-being.

No scientific studies have proven whether reiki is effective for treating any type of disease. But some health professionals believe it may be useful in helping reduce stress and anxiety.[144]

# References

## Chapter 1. Introduction

1. The World Health Report 1997, WHO, Report of the Director General, WHO
2. Love, S. Dr Susan, Love's Breast Book (2nd edition), Reading, MA: Addision-Wesley, 1995:24-25and 252-253.
3. John, L. Coscia, M.D. Breast Radiologist: Breast Health, Breast Care Centre of Texas, PA: from website
4. 50 years of cancer control in India, National Cancer Control Programme, DGHS, Ministry of Health and Family Welfare, Government of India, Nov 2002
5. Parkin, D M, Pisani F, Ferlay J (1999). Global cancer statistics, CA, Jan-Feb 49, 1
6. The World Health Report 1997, WHO, Report of the Director General, WHO
7. Ferlay, J, Bray, F, Pisani, P, Parkin, DM. GLOBOCAN 2002. Cancer Incidence, mortality and prevelance world-wide IARC Cancer base no. 5, Lyon, France, IARC Press 2004
8. Botha J. I, Bray F, Sankila R, Parkin, D M. Breast Cancer Incidence and mortality trends in 16 European coun-tries. European J Cancer 2003, 39:1718-29
9. National Cancer Registry Programme. Five year consolidated Report of the Hospital Based Cancer Registries 1994-1998, ICMR, Delhi, 2002.

10. National Cancer Registry Programme. Two Year Report of the Population Based Cancer Registries consoli-dated report 2001-03, ICMR, New Delhi
11. Sutirho, P. : Delhi, Mumbai Life Style Supports Breast Cancer Risk: Hindustan Times, July 22, 2002.
12. Balakrishna, B, Yeole, Kurkure, A.P (2003). An epidemiological assessment of increasing incidence and trends in breast cancer in Mumbai and other sites in India, during the last two decades. Asian Pacific Journal of Cancer Prevention, vol 4, 55.

## Chapter 2. The need for Breast Self Examination (BSE)

13. Love, S, Lindsey, K., Dr Susan Love's Breast Book, 2nd ed. Reading, MA: Addison-Wesley, 1995; 25. Wellisch D, et al. Annals Behav Med 2001; 23(4).
14. John, L. Coscia: Breast Health, Breast Care Centre of Texas, PA: from website
15. Holy Name Breast Health Center-from www.holyname.org
16. Barron, H. LennerWhen statistics provide unsatisfying answers: revisiting the beast self examination con-troversy. CMAJ, Jan, 22, 2002; 166(2).
17. Auchincloss, H. How more women can be saved from dying of cancer of thebreast. Med. J. Record,1929; 130:446-9.
18. Proctor, R. N.: The Nazi War on Cancer, Priceton(N) : Princeton University Press; 1999.
19. Self exam of the breasts. Good Housekeeping. 1955, Nov; 32
20. A frank film helps detect breast cancer. LOOK, 1950, Dec19; 87.
21. Thorlakeson PHT, Professional and Public education on cancer, CMAJ, 1951; 64:344-5.
22. Reagan, L. J. Engendering the dreaded disease: Women, men and Cancer. Am. J. Pub. Health, 1997; 87:1779-87.

23. Slaughter, F.S. The new science of surgery, New York: Julian Messner, 1946

    Introduction and The Problem 203

24. Is there something you are forgetting to do? (pamphlet). Philadelphia(PA): American Cancer Society, 195516-18-4

25. Jan Sheehan: Lifesaving Breast Cancer News, from the Breast Cancer Action Saskatchewan newsletter, vol 9, number 2:2003-09-30.

26. Park's Textbook of Preventive and Social Medicine, 17th edition, M/s Banarsidas Bhanot Publishers, Jabalpur, 2002

27. Thomas, D.B, GaoDL ,Ray R Metal. Randomization and trial of BSE in Shanghai: final results . J. Natl. Cancer Inst. 2002, Oct2; 94(19):1445-57. newsletter, vol 9, number 2:2003-09-30.

28. Breast Self-Examination: An option for the Early Detection of Carcinoma. July 2nd, 2009 Mayo Clinic Staff, from www.Mayo Clinic. com.

29. American Cancer Society Guidelines for Breast Cancer Screening, Update, CA Cancer J Clinic, 2003; 53:141-169

## Chapter 3. Breast Cancer and those at Risk

30. Bailey and Love's Short Practice of Surgery, 23rd edition, Arnold International Students Edition, London: 2001.

31. Detailed Guide: Breast Cancer What Are the Risk Factors for Breast Cancer? Cancer Reference Information, American Cancer Society 09/18/2006

32. Dr. A. Heather Eliassen, Postmenopausal Weight Gain Increases Breast Cancer Risk JAMA 2006; 296: 193-201.

33. Anderson, G. L, Judd, H. L, Kaunitz, A. M, Barad, D. H, et al. Effects of estrogen plus progestin on gynecologic cancers and associated diagnostic procedures: The Women's Health Initiative randomized trial. JAMA.2003; 290(13):1739-174

34. Polly A. Marchbanks, Jill A. McDonald, Hoyt G. Wilson, etal Oral Contraceptives and the Risk of Breast Cancer The New England Journal of Medicine Volume 346:2025-2032 June 27, 2002 Number 26, 14
35. Rowan, T. Chlebowski, Zhao Chen, Garnet, L. Anderson et al Ethinicity and breast cancer:Factors influencing differences and outcome. J. Nat Cancer Institute, Vol 97. No. 6, 2005.
36. Regina, G. Ziegler Anthropometry and Breast Cancer1 The Journal of Nutrition Vol. 127 No. 5 May 1997, pp. 924S-928S
37. P. D. Darbre Underarm cosmetics and breast cancer Journal of Applied Toxicology Volume 23, Issue 2, Pages 89 – 95
38. Scott Davis, Dana K. Mirick, Richard G. Stevens Night Shift Work, Light at Night, and Risk of Breast Cancer Journal of the National Cancer Institute, Vol. 93, No. 20, 1557-1562, October 17, 2001
39. The Lesbian and Bisexual Women's Health Project funded by Health Canada and Status of Women Canada, and co-coordinated by the British Columbia Centre of Excellence for Women's Health.
40. Vilhjálmur Rafnsson, Hrafn Tulinius, Jón Gunnlaugur Jónasson and Jón Hrafnkelsson Risk of breast cancer in female flight attendants: a population-based study (Iceland) Cancer Causes and Control Issue: Volume 12, Number 2, February 2001, Pages: 95 - 101

## Chapter 4. Diet and Breast Cancer

41. Trans Fat Task Force. 'TRANSforming the Food Supply'. Retrieved on 2007-01-07
42. Hunter, JE (2005). 'Dietary levels of trans fatty acids' basis for health concerns and industry efforts to limit use'. Nutrition Research 25: 499–513
43. Innis, Sheila M and King, D Janette (1999). 'trans fatty acids in human milk are inversely associated with concentrations of

essential all-cis n-6 and n-3 fatty acids and determine trans, but not n-6 and n-3, fatty acids in plasma lipids of breast-fed infants'. American Journal of Clinical Nutrition 70 (3): 383–390

44. "What's in that French fry? Fat varies by city", MSNBC (2006-04-12). Retrieved on 7 January 2007. AP story concerning

45. Food and nutrition board, institute of medicine of the national academies (2005). Dietary Reference Intakes for Energy, Carbohydrate, Fiber, Fat, Fatty Acids, Cholesterol, Protein, and Amino Acids (Macronutrients). National Academies Press. pp. 424

46. Breast Cancer Risk Linked To Red Meat, Study Finds, Washington Post, 2005

47. Taylor, E.F, et al. Meat consumption and risk of breast cancer in the UK women's cohort study. British Journal of Cancer 2007; 96:1139-1146v

48. BCERF Fact Sheet #1, Phytoestrogens and the Risk of Breast Cancer

49. OHSU study shows four daily servings of fruits and vegetables reduce breast cancer risk by half Rachel MacK-night. Oregon Health and Science University 27-Oct-2003

50. Japanese researchers report in the International Journal of Cancer. SOURCE: International Journal of Can-cer, October 2008

51. Prior R, Wu X, Schaich K (2005). 'Standardized methods for the determination of antioxidant capacity and phenolics in foods and dietary supplements'. J Agric Food Chem 53 (10): 4290–302

52. Xianquan S, Shi J, Kakuda Y, Yueming J (2005). 'Stability of lycopene during food processing and storage'. J Med Food 8 (4): 413–22

53. Rodriguez-Amaya D (2003). 'Food carotenoids: analysis, composition and alterations during storage and processing of foods'. Forum Nutr 56: 35–7. PMID 15806788

54. Baublis, A, Lu C, Clydesdale F, Decker E (2000). 'Potential of wheat-based breakfast cereals as a source of dietary antioxidants'. J Am Coll Nutr 19 (3 Suppl)
55. 2008 Women and Environments International Magazine. via Pro Quest Information and Learning Company; Cancer News Breast

    Cancer: The Link with Pesticides Women and Environments International Magazine.
56. The Lancet 1998; 352; 1816-1820
57. 10 Overlooked Reasons to Quit Smoking. Nicotine Found to Accelerate Breast Cancer By Charlene Laino Web MD Feature 10 www.healthfully.org
58. Web MD Health News Posted: Tuesday, April 15 2008. 12:24 Excess Alcohol May Increase Breast Cancer Risk
59. Lee I and Oguma Y. Physical Activity. In: Schottenfeld, D and Fraumeni JF, editors. Cancer Epidemiology and Prevention. 3rd ed. New York: Oxford University Press, 2006
60. IARC Handbooks of Cancer Prevention, Volume 6: Weight Control and Physical Activity, 2002
61. Mc Tiernan A, editor. Cancer Prevention and Management through Exercise and Weight Control. Boca Ra-ton: Taylor and Francis Group, LLC, 2006
62. Breast Cancer More Aggressive in Obese Women, Study research from The University of Texas M. D. An-derson Cancer Center. Suggests ScienceDaily (May 13, 2008)

# Chapter 5. Anatomy, Physiology and Development of Breast

63. Anatomy of a Working Breast by Anna Edgar Sebring FL USAFrom: New Beginnings, Vol. 22 No. 2, March-April, pp. 44-50

64. Sadler, T.W. Langmans Medical Embryology. Philadelphia, Pennsylvania: Lippincott, Williams, and Wilkins, 2000
65. Love, S. and Lindsey, K. Dr Susan Love's Breast Book. New York, New York: Addison Wesley, 1995
66. Tanner, J.M, Davies PS. Clinical longitudinal standards for height and weight velocity for North American children. J Pediatr 1985; 107:317-29. Highly useful growth charts with integrated standards for stages of puberty
67. Hartmann, P.E. et al. Breast development and control of milk synthesis. Food Nutr Bull 1996; 17:292-304
68. Wilde, D. J. et al. Autocrine regulation of milk secretion by a protein in milk. Biochem J 1995; 305:51
69. Mohrbacher, N. and Stock, J. THE BREASTFEEDING ANSWER BOOK. Schaumburg, Illinois: La Leche League International Patnaik, P. Axillary and vulval breasts associated with pregnancy. Br J Obstetric Gynaecol 1978; 85:156-7
70. Kent, J. Physiology of the expression of breast milk, part 2. Presented at the Medela Innovations in Breast Pump Research Conference, Boca Raton, Florida, July 2002.

## Chapter 6. Estrogen and the Risk of Breast Cancer

71. Programme on Breast Cancer and Environmental risk factors, Fact Sheet #09 March 1998 Estrogen and Breast Cancer Risk: What Is The Relationship? Learning Resources Events and Conferences Maps and Stats Research Resources BCERF Research Prepared by Prepared by Rachel Ann Clark, M.S., Science Writer, BCERF Suzanne Snedeker, Ph.D., Research Project Leader, BCERF and Carol Devine, Ph.D, R.D. Education Project Leader, BCERF
72. Marchant, D. J. Benign breast disease. Obstet Gynecol Clin North Am. 2002; 29(1): 1-20

73. Klein, S. Evaluation of palpable breast masses. Am Fam Physician. 2005; 71(9): 1731-1738

## Chapter 7. Types of Breast Cancer

74. National Breast Cnacer organization, www.breastcancer.org, types of breast cancer, last modified 17th Nov 2008
75. www. Cancerhelp.org .uk, Types of breast cancer, 2009
76. www.imaginis.com, beningn breast conditions, july 2009

## Chapter 8. When and how to Perform Breast Self Examination (BSE)

77. American Cancer Association-Guidelines for Breast cancer detection. www.cancer.org. American Cancer Society. Cancer Facts and Figures 2009. Atlanta, Ga: American Cancer Society; 2009. Last Medical Review: 03/05/2008

    Last Revised: 05/21/2009
78. Breast Self-Examination: An option for the Early Detection of Carcinoma. Mayo Clinic Staff, Mayo Clinic. www.mayoclinic.com
79. Bailey and Love's Short Practice of Surgery, 23rd edition, Arnold International Student's Edition, Lon-don:2001
80. Bridget Murray: Vertical-strips method for breast self-exam uses 'touch intelligence' A psychologist's beha-vioral insight leads to a better way of finding breast lumps. American Psychological Association VOLUME 29, NUMBER 12 –December, 1998

## Chapter 9. How to Diagnose Breast Cancer

79. Bailey and Love's Short Practice of Surgery, 23rd edition, Arnold International Student's Edition, London: 2001
81. In-depth analysis of Breast Cancer: A detailed feature, Medindia.net

82. Web MD, August 2005. SOURCE: The American Cancer Society
83. BC Cancer agency Care and Research www.bccancer.bc.ca

## Chapter 10. Pregnancy and Breast Cancer

84. Hoover, H. C Jr. Breast cancer during pregnancy and lactation. Surg Clin North Am. 1990 Oct; 70(5):1151-63
85. Breast cancer and pregnancy www. imaginis. com Updated: November 13, 2007
86. Pregnancy and Breast Cancer, American Cancer Reference Information ACS www.Cancer.org Last Medical Review: 08/28/2009 Last Revised: 08/28/2009
87. www.breastcancer.org Page last modified on: July 10, 2008
88. Carcinoma breast in pregnancy and lactation Suhag Virender, Sunita BS, Singh Subhash Deptt. of Radiothe-rapy and Oncology, Govt. Medical College and Hospital, Chandigarh, India
89. Pregnancy after Breast Cancer Mary L. Gemignani, MD, and Jeanne A. Petrek, MD From the Breast Service, Department of Surgery, Memorial Sloan-Kettering Cancer Center, New York, NY. www.moffitt.org
90. Breast Cancer in pregnancy,Breast Cancer Agency from website Updated: November 2004

    www.bccancer.bc.ca
91. Diagnosis and management of breast problems during pregnancy and lactation.Carol EH Scott-Conner, MD, PhD. Department of Surgery The University of Iowa Hospitals and Clinic

## Chapter 11. Types of Treatment

92. A Test of Time: Breast Cancer Awareness and Treatment through the Ages: WOMEN'S HEALTH.

    Rx.Magzaine, Story by Leah Shafer, April 2, 2002

93. Detailed Guide: Breast Cancer Surgical Procedures for Breast Cancer ACS, updated 9/2/5
94. Treatments and side effects. www.breastcancer.org Page last modified on: February 17, 2009

## Chapter 12. Side Effects of Treatment of Breast Cancer

95. Published by BUPA's Health Information Team, February 2004, Cancer treatment is either local therapy or systemic therapy:
96. Lymphodema after breast cancer surgery Side Effects of Treatment: Lymph edema www.MYWEBMD.com Web MD Medical Reference provided in collaboration with the Cleveland Clinic Edited by Paul O'Neill, MD on September 01, 2006

## Chapter 13. Evidence Based Management of Patients

97. Breast Cancer Guidelines Evidence-Based Management for Breast Cancer Evidence based guidelines: Tata Memorial Cancer Hospital, Mumbai from www.tatamemorialcentre.com

## Chapter 14. Issues after Breast Cancer Treatment

98. Detailed guide: breast cancer what happens after breast cancer treatment? American Cancer Society www.cancer.org Last Medical Review: 09/04/2008, Last Revised: 05/13/2009
99. Mary, L. Gemignani, MD, and Jeanne, A. Petrek, MD. Pregnancy after breast cancer, www.moffitt.org
100. Pregnancy after breast cancer: John, Hopkins gynecologic oncology, www.hopkinsmedicine.org

## Chapter 15. What is Counseling?

101. Living with Cancer: What is Counseling? Cancer research U.K, Last updated 6.9.2005

102. Breast Cancer Resource Guide of Connecticut UCc Con health center Neag Comprehensive Health Centre from www. Cancer. udhc.edu

103. Dharmen Patel, Lawrence Shapiro, and Robert G. Lerner, Genetic Counseling and Breast Cancer

104. Daniel Harber, MD, PhD: Editorials: Prophylactic Oophorectomy to reduce the risk ovarian and Breast cancer in carriers of BRCA mutation: New Engl. J Med, Vol. 346, No.21, 1660-1662, 2002

105. Am. J. Human Genet. 62:676-689, 1998

106. Journal of Clinical Oncology 17:3396-3402, 1998

107. Journal of National Cancer Institute 91:1310-1315, 1999

108. Ramus St et al. Nature Genetics 15:14-15, 1997

109. ND Kauff et al. Risk reducing salpingo-oophorectomy in carriers of BRCA1 or BRCA2 mutations:N Engl J Med, vol. 346, No. 21, 1616-1622, 2002

110. TR Rebbeck et al.Prophylactic oophorectomy in carriers of BRCA1or BRCA2 mutations: N Engl J Med, Vol 346, no 21, 1616-1622, 2002

111. Yang H, Jeffery, P. D, Miller J, Kinnucan E et al BRCA2 function in DNA binding and recombination from BRCA2-DSSI-ssDNA structrure. Science 2002, sept 13; 297(5588):1837-48

112. Elizabeth, G. Eakin, PhD, and Lisa A. Strycker, MA, of the Oregon Research Institute. Counseling Services Underutilized by Cancer Patients journal Psycho-Oncology stated in Article date: 2001/03/13 in America CS News Letter

## Chapter 16. Recurrence of Breast Cancer

113. Breast Cancer Recurrence: The Cleveland Clinic Foundation from the website last reviewed 11/17/2003

114. Recurrence of breast cancer from www.imaginis.com Updated: July 28, 2008

## Chapter 17. Breast Cancer in Men

115. France, L., Michie, S., Barrett Lee, P., Brain, K., Harperand, P., Gr, J., Male Cancer: A qualitative study of male breast cancer. The Breast (2000), 9: 343-348
116. Cancer Research UK 2002, Male Breast Cancer
117. Rai B, Ghoshal, S, Sharma, S.C. Breast cancer in males: A PGIMER experience. J Can Res Ther 2005; 1:31-33
118. Bose, S.M. ABC of Breast Cancer in the Sunday Tribune
119. Robert Preidt Health Scouts: Men usually slow to detect breast cancer, Scout's News, 6/2/2003
120. The Oston Globe (Washington) Men With Breast Cancer Go Public August 7, 2002
121. Breast Cancer in Men: www.Imaginis.Com (source:American cancer society) Updated: January 29, 2008
122. Breast Cancer in Men: National Cancer Resource Center

## Chapter 18. Alternative Therapies for Breast Cancer Treatment

123. Eisenberg, D, Kessler, R, Foster C, et al: Unconventional medicine in the United States: Prevalence, costs, and patterns of use. N Engl J Med 328: 246-252, 1993
124. Cassileth, B, Chapman C: Alternative and complementary cancer therapies. Cancer 77: 1026-1034, 1996.
125. National Center for Complementary and Alternative Medicine: Expanding Horizons of Healthcare: Five-Year Strategic Plan 2001-2005. Bethesda MD, Department of Health and Human Services and National Institutes of Health, 2000

126. What Is Complementary and Alternative Medicine? National Center for Complementary and Alternative Medicine: http://nccam.nih.gov/. Last Updated: 05/14/2008

127. Richardson MA, Sanders T, Palmer JL, et al: Complementary/alternative medicine use in a comprehensive cancer center and the implications for oncology. J Clin Oncol 18: 2505-2514, 2000.

128. Kaptchuk, T. J, Eisenberg, D. M: The persuasive appeal of alternative medicine. Ann Intern Med 129: 1061-1065, 1998

129. Patient decision-making about complementary and alternative medicine in cancer management: context and process L.G. Balneaves, RN PhD, * L. Weeks, † and D. Seely, ND MSc‡ Curr Oncol. 2008 August; 15(s2): s94–s100. 130. Yoga shown to reduce pain, fatigue in women with breast cancer Wednesday, October 10, 2007 by: David Gutierrez, staff writer

131. Yoga Helps Breast Cancer Patients: Eases Nausea, Improves Well-Being By Peggy Peck Web MD Health News SOURCE: American Society of ClinicalOncology, 39th Annual Meeting, Chicago, Illinois, May 31-June 3, 2003, 'Randomized Controlled Trial of Yoga for Symptom Management During Breast Cancer Treatment'

132. Restorative Yoga for Symptom Management and Stress Reduction in Women with Ovarian Cancer and Breast CancerWake Forest University Baptist Medical Center Principal Investigator:Suzanne C. Danhauer, Ph.D

133. Eur J Cancer Care 16:462-474, 2007 AMSA EDCAM INITIATIVE: A National Curriculum For Medical Students

134. Traditional Chinese Medicine, Kampo, Tibetan Medicine, and Acupuncture Authors: James E. Williams, OMD; Shan Liang, OMD; Efrem Korngold, OMD; Joseph Helms, MD

135. Janelle Wheat, Geoff Currie: Herbal medicine for cancer patients: An evidence based review. The Internet Journal of Alternative Medicine. 2008. Volume 5 Number 2

136. Traditional Chinese Medicine (TCM) in the Management of Gynecological cancers. XY Zhang, PhD, MD. Women's Health Clinic, London, UK

137. Estrogen Dependent Tumors And Herbs: How Modern Conditions Change Traditional Practices essay by Subhuti Dharmananda, Ph.D., Director, Institute for Traditional Medicine, PortlandOregon

138. Hatha Yoga: Its Context, Theory and Practice By Mikel Burley, Vedic books

139. Zen Buddhism: A History (India and China) By Heinrich Dumoulin, James W. Maison, A.; Herbert, J.R.; Werheimer, M.d.; and Kabat-Zinn, J. (1995). 'Meditation, melatonin and breast/prostate cancer: hypothesis and preliminary data,'. Medical Hypotheses 44 (1): 39–46

140. Maison, A.; Herbert, J.R.; Werheimer, M.d.; and Kabat-Zinn, J. (1995). "Meditation, melatonin and breast/prostate cancer: hypothesis and preliminary data,". Medical Hypotheses 44 (1): 39–46

141. Carlson, L.E, Ursuliak Z, Goodey E, Angen M, Speca M. (2001) The effects of a mindfulness meditation-based stress reduction program on mood and symptoms of stress in cancer outpatients: 6-month follow-up.

142. Care Cancer. 2001 Mar; 9(2):112-23. 143. Chant 'Om' for Better Heart Health. Monday, August 07, 2006 by: Natural News, Monday, August 07, 2006 by: Natural News, citizen journalist

143. Chant 'Om' for Better Heart Health. Monday, August 07, 2006 by: Natural News, Monday, August 07, 2006 by: Natural News, citizen journalist

144. Pain management: Reiki from www.WebMD.com, Last Updated: June 27, 2007